D1161035

K.-D. Wolff · F. Hölzle

Raising of Microvascular Flaps

A Systematic Approach

Second Edition

With 139 Figures and 58 Drawings

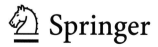 Springer

Prof. Dr. Dr. K.-D. Wolff
Technische Universität München
Klinikum rechts der Isar
Klinik und Poliklinik für
Mund-, Kiefer- und Gesichtschirurgie
Ismaninger Straße 22
81675 München
Germany
wolff@mkg.med.tum.de

Priv.-Doz. Dr. Dr. Frank Hölzle
Technische Universität München
Klinikum rechts der Isar
Klinik und Poliklinik für
Mund-, Kiefer- und Gesichtschirurgie
Ismaninger Straße 22
81675 München
Germany
hoelzle@mkg.med.tum.de

IV

ISBN 978-3-540-93831-6   eISBN 978-3-642-13831-7

DOI 10.1007/978-3-642-13831-7

Springer Heidelberg Dordrecht London New York

Library of Congress Control Number: 2011928507

© 2005, 2011 Springer-Verlag Berlin Heidelberg

This work is subject to copyright. All rights are reserved, whether the whole or part of the material is concerned, specifically the rights of translation, reprinting, reuse of illustrations, recitations, broadcasting, reproduction on microfilm or in any other way, and storage in data banks. Duplication of this publication or parts thereof is permitted only under the provisions of the German Copyright Law of September 9, 1965, in its current version, and permission for use must always be obtained from Springer-Verlag. Violations are liable for prosecution under the German Copyright Law.

The use of general descriptive names, trademarks, etc. in this publication does not imply, even in the absence of a specific statement, that such names are exempt from the relevant protective laws and regulations and therefore free for general use.

Product liability: The publishers cannot guarantee the accuracy of any information about dosage and application contained in this book. In every individual case the user must check such information by consulting the relevant literature.

Cover design: eStudio Calamar, Figueres/Berlin

Illustrator: Harald Konopatzki, Heidelberg

Printed on acid-free paper

Springer is part of Springer Science+Business Media (www.springer.com)

This book is dedicated to those
who put their bodies at the disposal
of teaching and science in medicine

Preface

With the introduction of microvascular tissue transfer in the early 1970s, a new universe of reconstructive possibilities was opened. In the meanwhile, this technique has proven to be one of the most important developments for our patients. One of the reasons for this triumphal march of reconstructive microsurgery is the high number of excellent textbooks describing all the numerous flaps that can be raised from nearly every region of the human body. Even though much high-level literature was already available, we gained very positive feedback and encouragement with the first edition of this book and we were asked to apply this concept to the next generation of flap raising, i.e., perforator flaps.

Thus we continued with high-quality photographs taken from clearly dissected sites that were split into a series of exactly defined sequences of flap elevation. Important anatomical landmarks and structures were explained, and a system in flap raising became obvious. This system has been developed in our courses over the last two decades during which we have instructed almost 1,000 colleagues from all over the world. This system has turned out to be extremely helpful not only in improving the understanding of the regional anatomy, but also in increasing the safety and success of flap raising.

The decisive stimulus to our book was provided by the opportunity to use cadavers that had been embalmed following Thiel's method. As can be seen from his brilliant photographic atlas, this embalming method provides excellent conditions for carrying out anatomical dissections. Thus, we decided to perform flap-raising procedures on this bloodless tissue. Moreover, the Thiel fixation method provided us with our first opportunity to shoot flap-raising video films without the usual restrictions of a sterile OR and the disadvantages of bleeding and poor visualization of the site. The operative techniques and order of the individual steps we describe are based on clinical experience and recognition of the typical failures and difficulties that have occurred during our flap-raising courses. Although various techniques, strategies, and approaches have proven useful at the different donor sites, we decided to focus solely on one standard procedure for each flap. These standard procedures represent the best combination of safety, simplicity, and reliability and can be varied or expanded as soon as the surgeon has gained sufficient experience. To meet the demand of readily available, precise, and comprehensive information, instruction on flap raising is mainly given by anatomical photographs and schematic drawings. The aim of the text is to describe the development, indications, anatomy, advantages, and disadvantages of all routinely used standard or perforator flaps. The complex surgical procedure of flap raising has been split into simple steps, making it much easier to end every operation successfully. This step-by-step strategy enhances the teaching character of this book. We also found it necessary to give a brief introduction of microvascular tissue transfer in general and to point out the development, definition, and classification of perforator flaps for a better understanding of these innovative flaps. Additionally, the videos that follow the same system and surgical techniques described in the book are intended to help the surgeon prepare for flap raising.

Every operation needs an aim and a plan. The aim is to help use proper indications that meet with the individual needs of every patient according to our best medical knowledge. For us as surgeons, the plan is the anatomy, which we must understand thoroughly and comprehensively, so that it can guide us straightforwardly during our work, leaving as little damage to the body as possible.

We hope this book will add further stimulus to learning the techniques of flap raising and will contribute to making microvascular tissue transfer an attractive and comprehensible method for all surgeons who are involved in oncology and reconstructive surgery.

Klaus-Dietrich Wolff

Acknowledgements

This second edition would not have been possible without the help and valuable support of some good friends and esteemed colleagues. First of all, we would like to thank the anatomists, who offered us the opportunity to run our flap-raising courses and perform all the dissections on cadavers. In this respect, we are extremely grateful to Prof. Graf and Prof. Bogusch from Charité Berlin, Prof. Dermietzel from Ruhr University Bochum, and Prof. Putz from Ludwig Maximilian University of Munich. The willingness of these anatomists to open the doors of their institutes to clinicians led to interesting events with fruitful discussions and was the inspiration for many participants to carry out further anatomical studies in order to answer specific clinical questions. The increasing demand for our courses has proven just how important they are in maintaining and improving our knowledge of human anatomy. The embalming procedures for the cadavers, performed professionally by Claudia Schneider and Helmut Riese in Bochum and Axel Unverzagt in Munich, and who were always friendly and helpful, were decisive in the quality of the photographs and videos. Harald Konopatzki provided us with excellent schematic drawings for teaching. His insight into anatomy, his experience as an illustrator, and his artistic talent enabled him to realize our ideas and wishes. This ability was excellent in the first edition and was perfected by means of his illustrations of the added perforator flaps in the second edition. It was a pleasure to work with him. We are also very grateful to Andreas Beyna, Dr. Florian Bauer, and Dr. Jochen Weitz who shot the videos and processed and improved the photographs of the cadaver preparations. Their professional knowledge made an important contribution to the quality of the figures and videos. Moreover, we would also like to express our gratitude to Springer-Verlag, especially Ms. Martina Himberger and Ms. Irmela Bohn, for all the useful advice and professional and reliable realization of this project. We thank Linda Northrup for reading and improving the manuscript. We would also like to thank Mr. David Mitchell, who has contributed with his outstanding clinical experience to the success of our courses since the early millennium and who has in the meantime become a good friend.

However, most of our gratitude goes to our families, our dear wives and children, who have shown virtually endless patience and understanding for our work. With their love, whole-hearted support, and cheerful natures, they have always been able to give us new energy; for this reason, they deserve the highest respect for the completion of this book.

The authors

Contents

Introduction

At the end of the nineteenth century, the first experimental and clinical work on the suturing of blood vessels was published by Murphy, who in 1897 performed the first end-to-end anastomosis in a human blood vessel [276]. Shortly thereafter, Carrel and Guthrie did experimental work on free tissue transfer in dogs using vascular anastomoses [53, 128], which later was awarded with the Nobel prize. With the introduction of the operating microscope by Nylen in 1921 [285], this pioneering work opened the door to microvascular surgery. Nevertheless, until the beginning of the 1960s safe and reliable suturing of blood vessels smaller than 2 mm in diameter was still impossible. After preparatory work on coronary vessels in dogs, it was Seidenberg who in 1958 replaced the carcinomatous part of a human esophagus with a tubed segment of the jejunum by means of microvascular anastomoses and thus performed the first free tissue transfer [345]. With further technical improvement of operating microscopes and refinements of suturing materials and needles, in 1960 Jacobson and Suarez were able to safely unify small vessels only 1 mm in diameter [174]. Within a few years, a number of publications appeared demonstrating the tremendous possibilities that were opened up by the technique of microvascular anastomoses in clinical practice, such as the first replantation of fingers by Kleinert and Kasdan [197] in 1963 and amputated arms by Malt and McKhann in 1964 [231]. Moreover, experimental research on composite-free tissue transfer for defect cover was done by Krizek and co-workers, and the first clinical case was published in 1971 by Antia and Buch, who raised a free dermis–fat flap pedicled at the superficial epigastric artery and vein for covering a skin defect on the face [11]. In the same year, Black and co-workers performed a palatal reconstruction using a jejunal flap [30], and McLean and Buncke covered a scalp defect with a flap from the omentum in 1972 [256]. Also in 1972, a cutaneous flap, which later developed to become the first standard flap, was introduced by McGregor and Jackson [255]. This groin flap, whose anatomy was further described by Daniel and Taylor [86, 87], soon was used for numerous reconstructive purposes until it was increasingly replaced by other flaps, particularly the radial forearm flap, which had vascular pedicles that made them more suitable for microvascular surgery. Additional improvement was provided by the work of Acland, who, in collaboration with industry, continuously developed and refined instruments and suturing materials for microvascular surgery [2, 3]. Since these first and fundamental steps, microvascular tissue transfer has made enormous progress, which mainly was driven by the desire to define ideal donor sites for any reconstructive problem. Among the many clinicians who made significant contributions to the development of new flaps and the understanding of their vascular anatomy, the name of Ian Taylor has to be mentioned first and foremost. With the numerous proven flaps developed thus far, today's choice of the appropriate donor site seems to be more difficult than the reconstruction itself.

Radial Forearm Flap

1

Wolff/Hölzle, *Raising of Microvascular Flaps 2nd ed.*,
DOI: 10.1007/978-3-642-13831-7_1, © Springer-Verlag Berlin Heidelberg 2011

Development and Indications

In 1978, a fasciocutaneous free flap from the volar aspect of the forearm and pedicled on the radial artery was first used in China. When this so-called Chinese flap was originally described by Yang et al. in 1981 [440] and Song et al. in 1982 [360], both groups already had performed more than 100 successful flap transfers. Shortly thereafter, this technique was popularized by different European surgeons, who visited their colleagues in China. In 1981, Mühlbauer was the first to describe the advantages of the radial forearm flap in the European literature, especially its excellent pliability, thinness, the ease of flap raising, as well as the constant anatomy and the long and high-caliber vascular pedicle [271, 272]. Very soon, many authors favored this flap for reconstructions in the head and neck region and for intraoral lining. In a number of publications, Soutar and co-workers reported on different indications of the radial forearm flap for reconstructions of the oral cavity and the hand [362–365], and Cheng used this flap for tongue reconstruction [65]. Hatoko et al. and Chen et al. favored the forearm flap for defect coverages in the hard and soft palate and proposed this flap for the rehabilitation of the cleft lip and palate patient [62, 144]. Apart from a reliable closure of oroantral fistulas, they where able to resurface the alveolar ridge and to build a vestibule for reliable fitting of dentures. Moreover, the forearm flap was used as a tubed flap to reestablish the ability of phonation or deglutition by inserting it in defects of the hypopharynx, trachea, or esophagus [61, 141, 439]. By including a bony segment of the radius, an osteocutaneous flap can be raised, which was proposed for mandible reconstruction [271, 363, 367]. Because of the rich vascularization, two ore more isolated skin paddles can be built, which are suitable for closure of perforating defects of the oral cavity [40]. Niranjan and Watson described a technique for cheek reconstruction using the tendon of the palmaris longus muscle to elevate the denervated angle of the mouth [283]. Lip reconstructions were performed by incorporating a segment of the brachioradialis muscle into the radial flap, which was then reinnervated by a branch of the facial nerve and sutured to the ends of the resected orbicularis muscle [323, 373]. As another variation, vascularized fascial flaps from the forearm were placed in the oral cavity to allow for re-epithelialization and thus to achieve a mucosal surface [239]. When covering the fascia with a skin graft prior to flap raising, ultrathin flaps can be prefabricated, which show less shrinkage compared to pure fascial flaps. Moreover, the appearance of the donor site is improved by linear closure of the forearm skin, which is not used for flap raising [428]. Although sensory recovery of the radial forearm flap may be facilitated by anastomosing a branch of the antebrachial cutaneous nerve to a sensory nerve of the recipient site [400], clinical experience has shown that sensation will at least partially be reestablished spontaneously after several years even without neurocutaneous anastomoses, probably by nerve sprouting. Apart from these many indications in the head and neck area, the radial forearm flap is a workhorse flap in traumatology of the extremities and trunk and may be used in many other reconstructive procedures.

Anatomy

The radial artery, which forms the deep palmar arch at the hand, is located in the lateral intermuscular septum between the brachioradialis and flexor carpi radialis muscles, giving off 9–17 branches to the forearm fascia [399], most of them existing in the distal third of the forearm. The strongest of these branches, the cubitalis inferior artery, is located proximally at the forearm [350, 399]. These numerous fascial branches form a dense fascial plexus that provides perfusion of the entire forearm skin. This makes the forearm flap a fasciocutaneous flap. Although the radial artery, which terminates in the deep palmar arch, is the main source vessel for the cutaneous branches of the forearm, the ulnar artery as well as the anterior and posterior interosseous arteries contribute to the blood supply of the forearm skin and the hand as well [72, 74]. According to a clinical study by Kerawala, the arterial backflow pressure of the distal stump of the radial artery is a mean 40 mmHg [183]. Thus, the vascular supply to the hand is normally maintained, and ischemia of the hand after raising the radial flap [164] as well as vascular anomalies, such as duplication of the of the radial artery [238, 331] or other irregularities [358], are very seldom described. A number of unnamed branches of the radial artery to the skin, muscles, and periosteum enable the transfer of different flap types with a great variety in design and flap components. Having in mind that the entire skin of an amputated forearm can safely be transferred at the radial artery alone [399], the size of the flap can vary considerably. Song and Gao pointed out that all cutaneous vessels travel with the antebrachial fascia, most of them between the brachioradialis and flexor carpi radialis muscles at the distal third of the forearm [360]. Therefore, the forearm fascia must be left attached to the undersurface of the skin during flap raising. Nutrition of the bone is provided by periosteal and direct medullar as well as indirect vascular branches, which perforate the flexor pollicis longus muscle and anastomose with the medullary vascular system. Alternatively, the forearm skin can be transferred at the ulnar or cubitalis inferior artery, designing the skin paddle over the ulnar side of the forearm. Given that the ulnar skin is less hair-bearing, the ulnar forearm flap was considered to be of higher skin quality [217], leading to lower donor site morbidity when raised at the proximal part of the forearm [226]. A disadvantage of the ulnar forearm flap is that it carries a significantly smaller number of cutaneous branches. According to Morrison, cutaneous branches from the ulnar artery can be missing completely [268]. Venous drainage of the forearm flap is established either by the deep radial veins or by the superficial venous system, which form multiple anastomoses between each other. Because of the different branching patterns of the deep and the superficial venous systems and the variability in the size and the course of the subcutaneous veins [387], the decision of whether to anastomose a superficial or deep vein has to be made on a case-by-cases basis. Although the large caliber of the subcutaneous veins makes for easier anastomosis, venous drainage by the superficial system can become unreliable in small flaps and after occult damage of the intima, for example caused by repeated catheterization of the vein.

Flow volumes of the superficial and deep veins were measured using Doppler ultrasonography, showing a significantly higher blood flow through the deep veins compared to the superficial veins in the early stage of flap transfer [168, 169]. Despite the presence of valves in the deep and superficial system, a retrograde flow is possible via the numerous interconnecting veins, making it possible to raise distally based radial forearm flaps [101, 222, 237, 388], which may be useful as pedicled flaps for defect cover of the hand [176].

Advantages and Disadvantages

The radial forearm flap is a thin, pliable, and mostly hairless fasciocutaneous flap, of great value for reconstructions in the head and neck region, especially in the oral cavity. The high caliber of the vessels (artery, 2–3 mm; cephalic vein, 3–4 mm; deep veins, 1–3 mm) and the long vascular pedicle as well as the variability in flap perfusion (ortho- and retrograde flow, venous drainage via the superficial or deep system) considerably facilitate anastomoses. Flap raising is possible simultaneous to tumor resection in the head and neck area and can be carried out quickly. Because of the ease of flap elevation, the radial forearm flap is recommended for beginners in free flap surgery. In addition to these advantages, some disadvantages have to be pointed out concerning the donor site of the forearm flap: because harvesting the flap always leads to complete interruption of the radial artery, perfusion of the hand must be maintained by the ulnar artery and the remaining anterior and posterior interosseous vessels. In an anatomic investigation on 750 cadavers, the radial and ulnar arteries were always found to be present, and the dominant vessel for hand perfusion was regularly found to be the ulnar artery, which terminates in the superficial palmar arch [252]. Nevertheless, blood supply to the thumb and index can totally depend on the integrity of the radial artery, if two anatomical variations coexist: first, if there are no branches of the superficial palmar arch to the index and thumb, and second, if there is no anastomosis between the deep and superficial palmar arch [78, 266]. To prevent postoperative ischemia of the hand, the Allen test or, if doubt persists, an angiography has to be carried out to prove the reliability of hand perfusion via the ulnar artery. Absence of the radial artery was described by Porter, who found the arterial supply of the forearm to be based on codominant median and ulnar arteries [295]. A considerable disadvantage is the appearance of the donor site, which is located in an esthetically exposed region. A number of publications can be found reporting on complications at the donor site, with a frequency of 30–50%, mostly caused by the poor transplant bed for the split-thickness skin graft [20, 41, 100, 105, 131–133, 242, 254, 362, 364, 370, 389]. To reduce donor site morbidity, different techniques have been developed to achieve direct wound closure, such as the V-Y plasty [100], the transposition flap [20], the use of tissue expanders [131, 242], or prelamination of the forearm fascia [428]. According to McGregor, harvesting the skin graft can be improved by bringing the wrist in an extended position for 20 days [254].

To achieve protection of the flexor carpi radialis tendon, it has been proposed to cover this tendon by oversewing it with the flexor muscles [105] or to provide a well-vascularized bed for the split-thickness skin graft by approximating the flexor digitorum muscle to the flexor and abductor pollicis longus muscles [198]. Apart from these problems concerning the healing of the donor site, other complications such as edema formation, reduced strength and extension of the hand, loss of sensitivity due to injury of the superficial branches of the radial nerve, and cold intolerance have been reported [389]. Following harvesting of an osteocutaneous forearm flap, the arm has to be immobilized for about 6 weeks; nevertheless, fractures are common [389], unless the donor arm is primarily stabilized by rigid plate fixation [409]. Using the tibia of sheep, Meland and co-workers found a considerable weakness and loss of stability of the bone even if only small amounts of the cortical bone have been removed [258]. Therefore, and because of other flaps available providing much more bone material to be raised, the osteocutaneous forearm flap cannot be considered a first-line method for mandible reconstruction. Finally, there is a tendency of edema formation in the flap, probably by changing the perfusion from a flow-through to a terminal-flow pattern. This edema can sometimes cause functional restrictions, especially in the oral cavity, but within a few weeks, it dissolves spontaneously [42]. Although the radial forearm flap is still a workhorse flap, especially in the head and neck area, these disadvantages may considerably reduce its acceptance among surgeons and patients [233].

Flap Raising

Preoperative Management

The Allen test has to be performed to assess the adequacy of the circulation of the hand (especially of the thumb) through the ulnar artery alone after sacrifice of the radial artery. Flap raising is carried out on the non-dominant arm (mostly on the left side). The use of a tourniquet is not mandatory, because with consequent hemostasis, the operating field can be held absolutely dry even in the perfused arm.

Patient Positioning

The arm is brought in an abduced and supine position so that the volar aspect of the entire forearm can be used for flap elevation. Circular disinfection is necessary from the fingers up to the axilla.

The distal flap border is placed 3 cm proximal to the wrist, and the ulnar margin of the flap is outlined over the flexor carpi ulnaris muscle. If the cephalic vein, which is variable in size and course and can be completely missing, is not used for venous drainage, the radial flap margin is placed over the brachioradialis muscle. The flap should not be extended to the dorsal aspect of the arm for aesthetic reasons. Drainage through the deep veins alone is always reliable and sufficient. The position of the proximal margin depends on the flap size needed. For exposure of the proximal vascular pedicle, a wave line incision helps to reduce postoperative scar shrinkage.

The skin is incised at the ulnar border through the subcutaneous fatty tissue until the forearm fascia is reached. The fascia, which has a dense and tight structure, is bluntly undermined above the flexor carpi ulnaris tendon.

Step 1

The fascia is incised and elevated, until the tendon of the flexor carpi ulnaris muscle is exposed. The paratenon, which envelopes the tendon, is left untouched. The cut margin of the fascia is clearly visible.

Step 2

The incision at the distal margin is made through the skin and the fascia in the same fashion. The flap, containing skin, subcutaneous tissue, and fascia can now be elevated. The further dissection is performed strictly underneath the fascia, and the tendons of the flexor digitorum and palmaris longus muscles become visible. The fibrous attachments between the undersurface of the forearm fascia and the paratenon are carefully transected. The paratenon itself is not removed. If, as in this case, the palmaris longus tendon is hypoplastic, it is transected and left attached to the fascia.

Step 3

6

Now the strong tendon of the flexor carpi radialis muscle is reached and subsequently isolated from the forearm fascia in its distal portion.

Step 4

Directly radial to this tendon, the radial artery is palpated, which runs into the septum between the flexor carpi radialis and brachioradialis muscles. At the most distal point, this septum is opened and a short segment of the radial artery is exposed. Before ligating the artery, which is always accompanied by two veins, the superficial branch of the radial nerve is identified over the tendon of the brachioradialis muscle. The nerve is carefully preserved during further dissection.

Step 5

The radial artery is divided at the distal border of the flap. In the perfused arm, the pulsation of the distal stump of the radial artery, caused by the intact circulation through the palmar vessel arches, is visible.

Step 6

Step 7

Now the skin incision is made 1 cm radial to the artery down to the forearm fascia. The cephalic vein and the superficial branches of the radial nerve are left intact. If the cephalic vein is included and used for venous drainage, the flap is extended towards the dorsal aspect of the forearm, and the cephalic vein is divided distally.

Step 8

The fascia is incised keeping a safe distance to the radial artery, and the tendon of the brachioradialis muscle is exposed and retracted laterally. Having identified the superficial branch of the radial nerve, the intermuscular septum, which contains the radial artery, is separated from the brachioradialis muscle. The artery is carefully elevated together with the flap and remains firmly connected to the forearm fascia. Numerous small branches to the deep muscles and the radial bone have to be cauterized or clipped in this area. The deep dissection plane during this step of flap raising is above the flexor pollicis longus muscle.

Step 9

It can be clearly seen that the undersurface of the flap is built by the forearm fascia and that the vascular bundle is securely attached to the fascia by the intermuscular septum. In the distal third of the forearm, where the radial artery is not covered by muscle bellies, the septum contains the highest number of cutaneous perforators. Because these perforators first reach the fascia to form a dense vascular network before they enter the skin, the radial forearm flap is a fasciocutaneous flap. The hypoplastic tendon of the palmaris longus muscle is left attached to the flap fascia and is removed from the forearm so that the skin graft takes well.

Step 10

Apart from the safe skin perfusion in this area, outlining the flap over the distal third of the forearm has the advantage of obtaining a long vascular pedicle. For dissection of the pedicle, the skin incision is made at the proximal border of the flap, where one or more cutaneous veins, which run superficial to the fascia, can be observed. If a vein is identified coming from the central part of the flap, it can be left intact for additional venous drainage. A wave-like skin incision is made for exposure of the proximal segment of the vascular pedicle.

Step 11

Prior to incision of the forearm fascia, the superficial cutaneous vein is traced proximally by careful subcutaneous dissection. To test the drainage adequacy, blood flow through this vein is observed by cutting it proximally at the end of flap raising before the radial artery is ligated. If there is adequate return of venous blood, the vein can be used as an additional drainage to the deep radial veins. By careful preparation, a cutaneous antebrachial nerve becomes visible, giving the opportunity to create a sensate flap.

The forearm fascia is now incised between the bellies of the brachioradialis and flexor digitorum muscles, and the vascular pedicle is exposed by retracting the brachioradialis muscle. It can clearly be seen that the septum between the brachioradialis and the flexor digitorum muscle has been removed from the distal third of the forearm, where the skin paddle was raised.

Step 12

The vascular pedicle is traced proximally so that sufficient length for a safe anastomosis is obtained. Although it is possible to dissect the pedicle up to the brachial artery, this is only rarely necessary. Excess pedicle length can lead to kinking of the pedicle at the recipient site and cause vascular occlusion. Careful hemostasis must be provided at the pedicle to prevent diffuse bleeding after opening the anastomoses.

Step 13

At the end of flap raising, residual connections between the flap and the flexor carpi radialis tendon are transected at the flap hilum, and the vascular pedicle is completely freed from the donor site. Ligation of the pedicle is not performed until the recipient vessels are ready for anastomosis.

Step 14

For reliable perfusion of the flap, anastomosing the radial artery and one of the deep radial veins is always safe and sufficient. Because the veins are closely connected to the artery and can be small in diameter, venous anastomosis requires microsurgical experience. The veins should be separated from the artery using the microscope. If a superficial vein is included, it can be used as additional venous drainage. The cephalic vein can be used as the only venous drainage when the flap has been extended to the dorsal aspect of the forearm so that it is safely located within the flap margins. If only a small flap is necessary, venous drainage through a cutaneous vein alone can become problematic because of the well-known anatomic variability of the superficial venous system.

Step 15

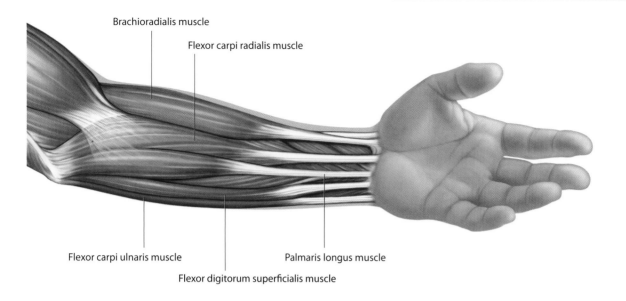

Brachioradialis muscle

Flexor carpi radialis muscle

Flexor carpi ulnaris muscle

Palmaris longus muscle

Flexor digitorum superficialis muscle

Flexor muscles of the forearm

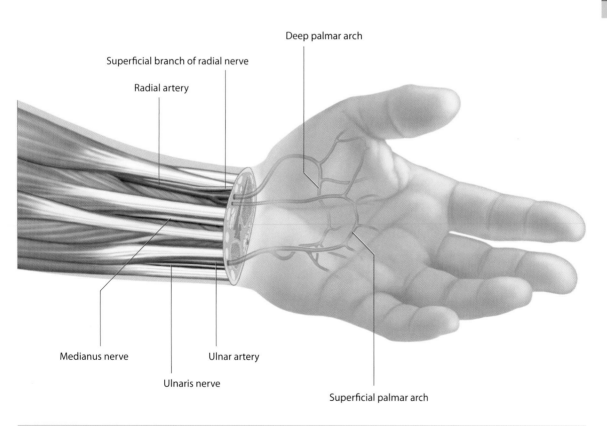

Deep palmar arch

Superficial branch of radial nerve

Radial artery

Medianus nerve

Ulnaris nerve

Ulnar artery

Superficial palmar arch

Vascular arches of the hand

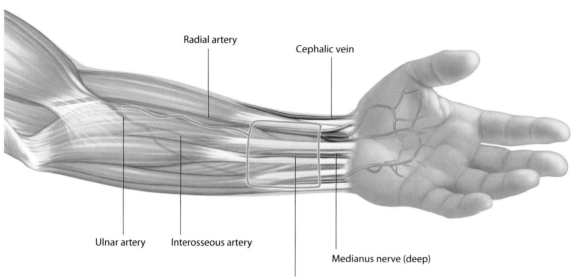

Radial artery

Cephalic vein

Ulnar artery

Interosseous artery

Medianus nerve (deep)

Medial antebrachial cutaneous vein

Standard flap design

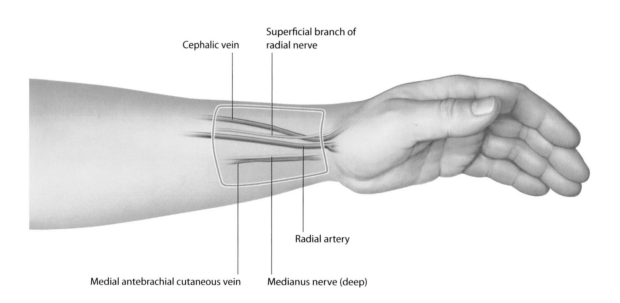

Cephalic vein

Superficial branch of radial nerve

Medial antebrachial cutaneous vein

Medianus nerve (deep)

Radial artery

Dorsal extension for inclusion of the cephalic vein

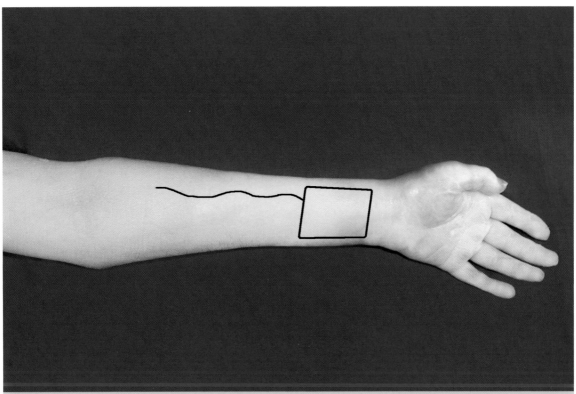

Standard design of the radial forearm flap

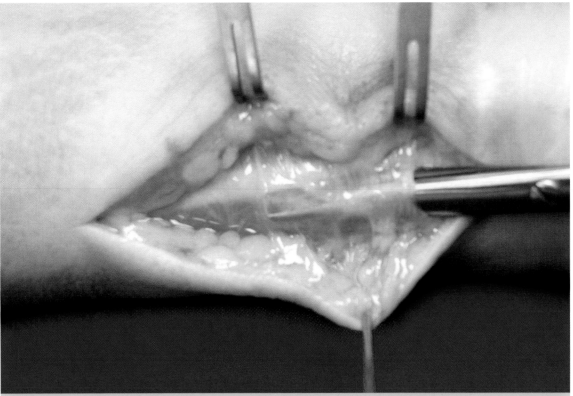

Step 1 • Ulnar skin incision and undermining of forearm fascia

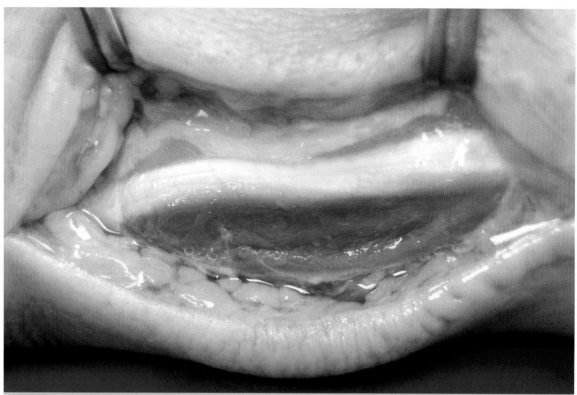

Step 2 • Incision of fascia and exposure of flexor carpi ulnaris

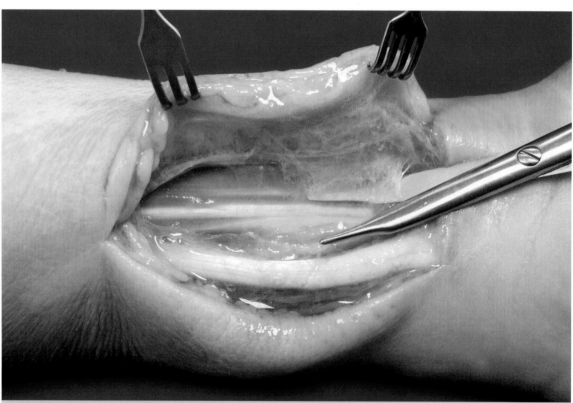

Step 3 • Distal skin incision, subfascial dissection

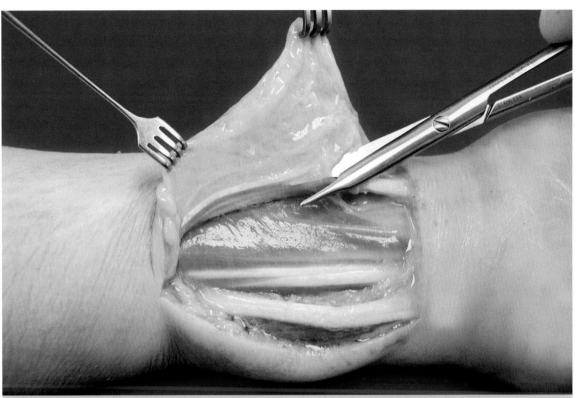

Step 4 • Exposure of the flexor carpi radialis tendon

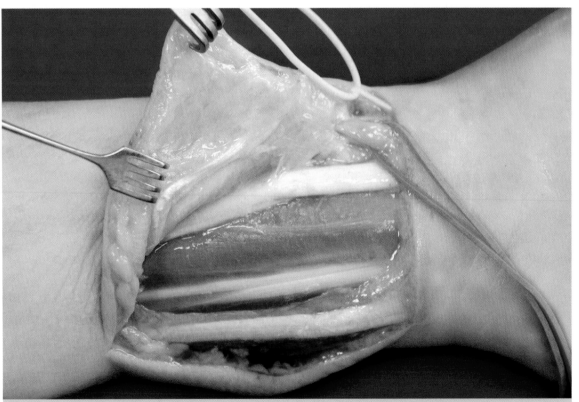

Step 5 • Identification of radial vessels and superficial radial nerve at distal flap margin

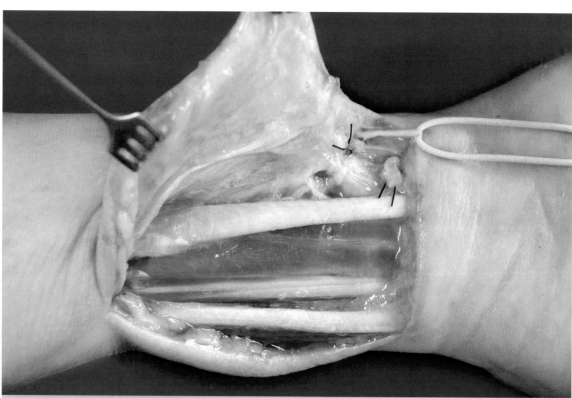

Step 6 • Ligation of radial vessels at distal flap border

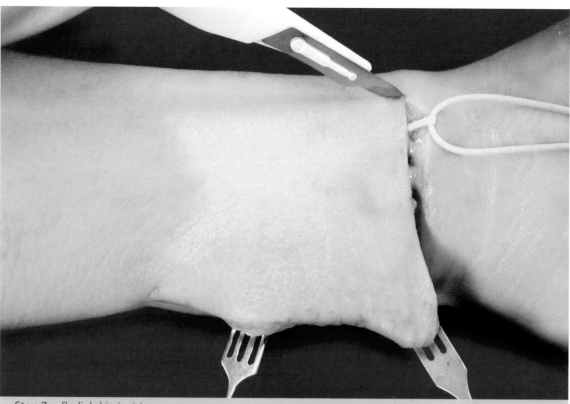

Step 7 • Radial skin incision

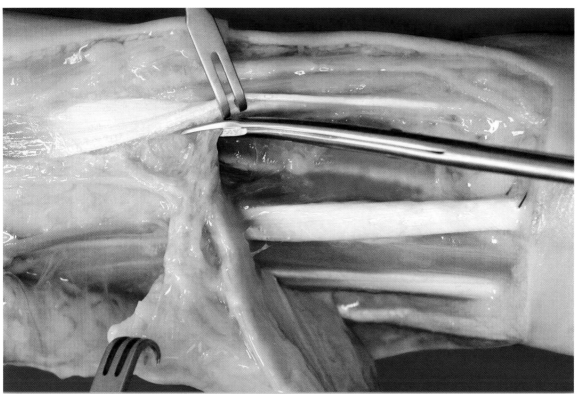

Step 8 • Dissecting the pedicle along brachioradialis muscle

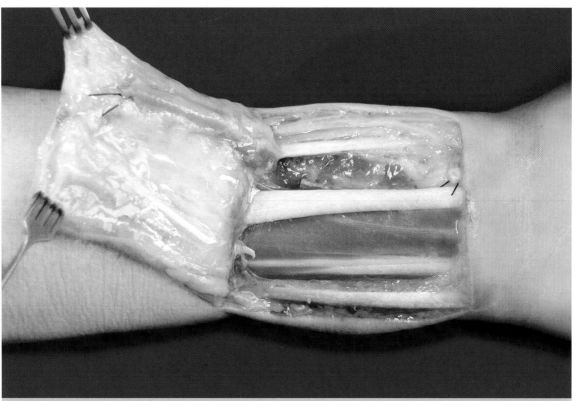

Step 9 • Complete subfascial flap elevation

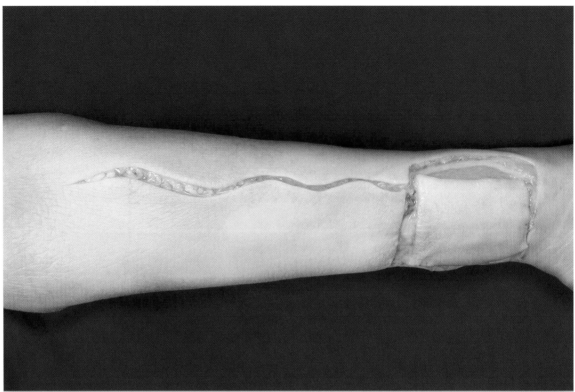

Step 10 • Skin incision at proximal flap margin and wavy incision for exposure of pedicle

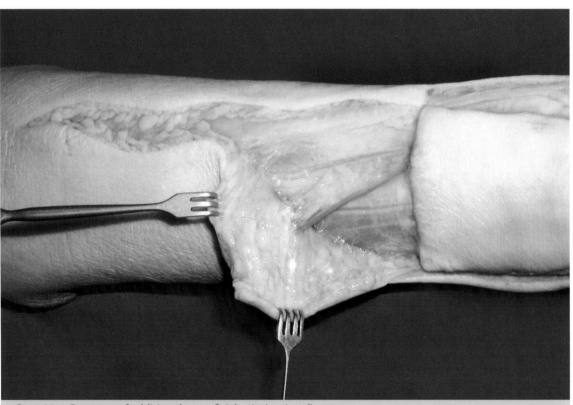

Step 11 • Exposure of additional superficial vein (optional)

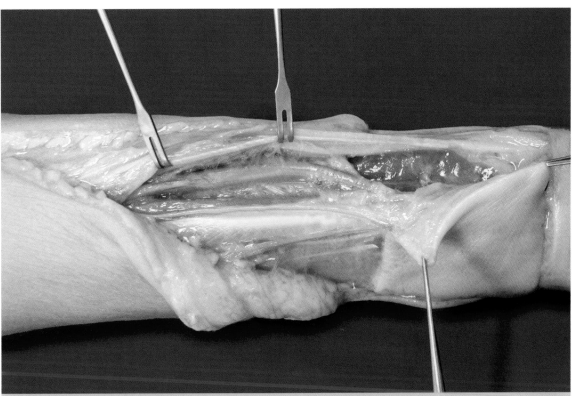

Step 12 • Exposure of vascular pedicle

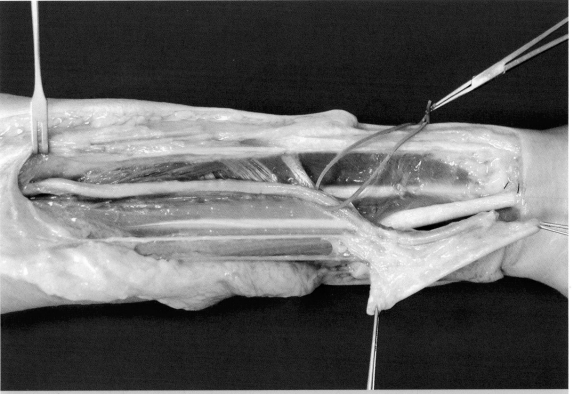

Step 13 • Complete dissection of pedicle

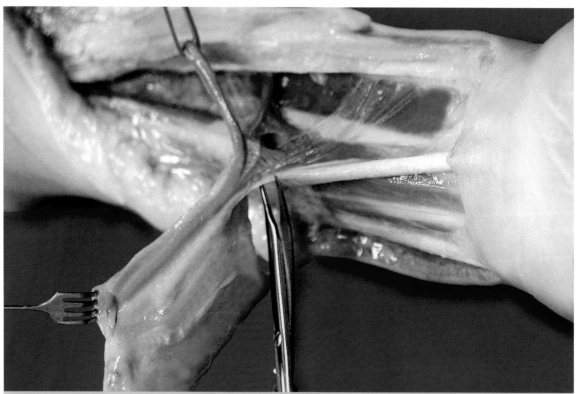

Step 14 • Separation of residual attachments at flap hilum

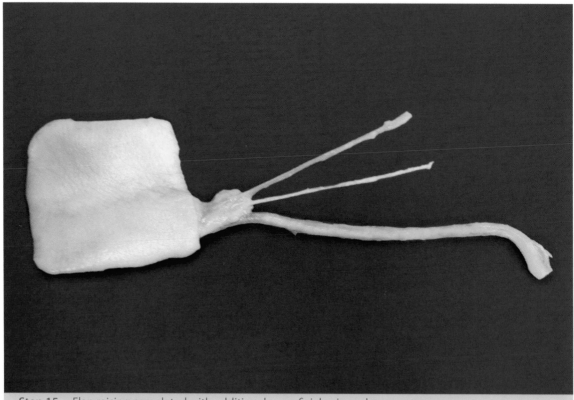

Step 15 • Flap raising completed with additional superficial vein and nerve

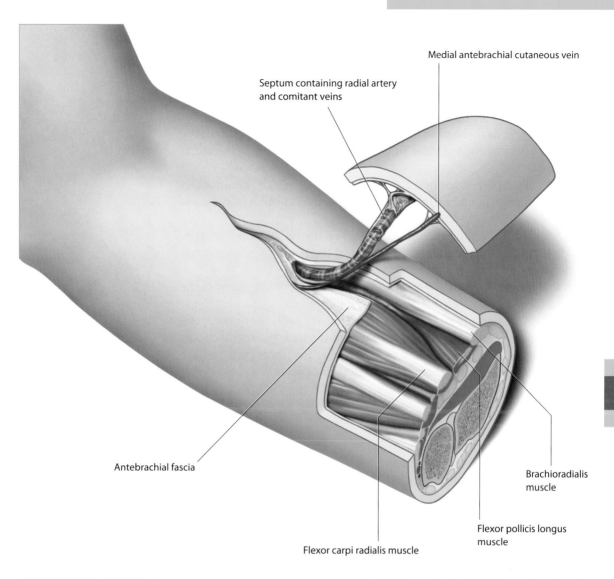

Medial antebrachial cutaneous vein

Septum containing radial artery and comitant veins

Antebrachial fascia

Flexor carpi radialis muscle

Flexor pollicis longus muscle

Brachioradialis muscle

19

Cross-section anatomy of left forearm

Comments

Step 2: To prevent an incorrect dissection plane above the fascia, incise the fascia, until the underlying muscle becomes clearly visible. We advise not dissecting deep to the flexor carpi ulnaris muscle to prevent injury to the ulnaris artery. As a variation, the ulnaris artery can run superficial to the muscle (the ulnaris pulse can be palpated). If the ulnar artery is violated, raise an ulnaris flap instead of using the radial vessels.

Step 3: We advise not removing the paratenon completely, because this will disturb wound healing. Fascia and paratenon can best be separated using a sharp scalpel.

Steps 5, 7: Injuring the superficial branch of the radial nerve is easily possible. In slim patients, the location of the nerve can be palpated through the skin.

Step 8: Injuring the vascular pedicle is possible in this step; retract the brachioradialis muscle for dissection of the pedicle.

Steps 10, 11: Choosing an insufficient superficial vein as the only venous drainage will lead to venous congestion of the flap. We advise checking the venous return of the superficial vein. The flexor carpi radialis tendon should be oversewn by muscle bellies so that the skin graft takes better.

Lateral Arm Flap

Wolff/Hölzle, *Raising of Microvascular Flaps 2nd ed.*,
DOI: 10.1007/978-3-642-13831-7_2, © Springer-Verlag Berlin Heidelberg 2011

Development and Indications

This first septocutaneous flap was originally introduced in 1982 by Song and co-workers [359] and 2 years later was described in more detail by Katsaros et al. [180]. Similar to the radial forearm flap, the lateral upper arm flap is relatively thin, but limited in width, and can be transferred together with a segment of bone, muscle, or sensory nerves. The flap, which is raised at the lateral aspect of the upper arm, is perfused by the terminal branches of the profunda brachii artery. This artery is not essential for the vascularity of the extremity. Early clinical series document a number of application possibilities, especially in the head and neck area [81, 82, 248, 344, 351, 412]. Because of its texture and the favorable color match, the flap is well suited for replacement of the facial skin [359]. At the extremities, the upper arm flap is useful for defect cover on the foot, hand, or forearm as a free flap [217, 268, 286, 338, 412] or as a pedicled flap for coverage of defects in the shoulder region [82, 412]. For defect cover in the temporal region, Inoue and Fujino left the flap pedicled on the cephalic vein, whereas the flap artery was microsurgically anastomosed to a neck artery [171]. Apart from these indications, the lateral upper arm flap can be used for a number of intraoral reconstructions. Matloub and co-workers reported on six reconstructions following partial or total glossectomy or defect cover at the hard palate [248]. By connecting the posterior cutaneous nerve of the arm to the lingual nerve, they were able to achieve neurocutaneous reinnervation. Including a cortical segment of the humerus, a limited amount of bone can be harvested together with the skin paddle, which was used for lower jaw reconstruction [248, 412]. Other authors confirmed the usefulness of the lateral upper arm flap for intraoral reconstructions in larger clinical series [73, 141, 304], especially the high success rate of neurocutaneous reinnervation after nerve coadaptation [73]. When extending the flap to the proximal forearm, the thin and pliable forearm skin can be combined with the thicker flap portion of the upper arm [73]. Moffett and co-workers demonstrated the possibility of dividing the flap, which then can be used for closure of through-and-through defects of the oral cavity [265].

Anatomy

The lateral upper arm flap is supplied by septocutaneous branches of the posterior radial collateral artery (PRCA), which develops from the profunda brachii artery. The cutaneous branches of the flap run within the lateral intermuscular septum, which separates the brachialis from the triceps muscle. According to Myong, the profunda brachii artery branches off from the brachialis artery as a singular vessel in 52% or together with the ulnar collateral artery in 30% of patients [277]. In 8%, the vessel was found to arise directly from the axillaris artery, and different studies describe a double profunda brachii artery with an incidence of 4–12% [180, 265, 311]. In these rare cases, each of the arteries has to be temporarily occluded to test their contribution to flap perfusion [265]. The proximal diameter of the artery varies from 0.9 to 2.5 mm [81, 180, 277], measuring 1.2 [248] or 1.5 mm on average [81, 180]. In close proximity to the radial nerve, the vascular pedicle spirals around the humerus, and proximal to the lateral intermuscular septum it divides into the small anterior and the stronger posterior radial collateral artery (PRCA). Whereas the small anterior radial collateral artery runs together with the radial nerve, the PRCA is the main nutrient artery of the flap, giving off the septocutaneous branches. After having traversed the septum at its base, the PRCA anastomoses with the interosseous recurrent artery, on which the flap can be perfused in a retrograde fashion. Because the proximal segment of the profunda brachii artery runs underneath the long and lateral head of the triceps muscle, dissection of the vascular pedicle to a proximal direction can be difficult. The average length of the pedicle that is not covered by the triceps muscle is 7–8 cm [248, 265]. By longitudinal splitting of the abovementioned triceps heads, the profunda brachii artery and veins can be followed up to the brachial vessels, obtaining a pedicle that is 6–8 cm longer [265]. It must be mentioned that this maneuver can reduce the strength of the operated arm, possibly following injury of muscular branches of the radial nerve [265]. The posterior cutaneous nerve of the arm (PCNA), which accompanies the PRCA and always has to be sacrificed during flap elevation, can be used to create sensate flaps [248, 286, 359, 412]. The posterior cutaneous nerve of the forearm (PCNF) does not provide sensation to the flap and could be preserved during flap elevation, but for technical reasons, this nerve is normally sacrificed as well. Venous drainage is most reliable by the comitant veins of the profunda brachii, because the cephalic vein mostly runs too far medially at the upper arm [286]. When outlining the skin paddle, the flap axis is positioned along the intermuscular lateral septum, which is defined by the interconnecting line between the lateral epicondyle and deltoid insertion. Although the skin territory can be as large as 18×11 cm [248], flaps should always be located within the safety zone, extending 12 cm proximal to the lateral epicondyle and including one-third of the circumference of the upper arm [311, 412]. According to anatomic studies using dye injections, the distal extension of the flap is possible up to 8 cm inferior of the lateral epicondyle [214]. Harvesting a cortical segment of humerus is technically possible, but only to a size of 10×1 cm, leaving a muscle cuff on either side of the septum to include periosteal vessels of the PRCA [81]. Direct closure of the donor site is only possible if the width of the flap does not exceed 6–7 cm. For aesthetic reasons, the use of a skin graft should be avoided in this area [286].

Advantages and Disadvantages

The lateral upper arm flap has a reliable and constant anatomy, and because of the good color match and similar texture, the flap is suitable for defect coverage on the face and neck. Compared to the radial forearm flap, raising this flap is technically more demanding because of the deeper location of the pedicle and its close relationship with the radial nerve. Although in normal-weight patients the flap carries only a thin layer of subcutaneous fat, the average thickness of the adipose layer is 1.3 cm [119], and a considerable amount of the subcutaneous fatty tissue can be found in adipose patients [286]. The possibility of creating sensate flaps is considered an advantage, especially in tongue reconstructions [248]. The combination of the skin paddle with a segment of the humerus bone or triceps muscle may contribute to a wider spectrum of indications for the flap [81, 180]. The high and reliable vascularity of the fascia allows for raising purely fascial flaps, which can be covered with split thickness skin grafts [359]. These fascial flaps have proven to be useful in reconstructions of the ear and nose [73]. The main disadvantage of the flap is the limited length of the pedicle and the small diameter of the vessels, so that anastomoses can become difficult, especially following radical neck dissection [265, 286, 412]. Flap raising leads to sensory loss at the proximal and posterior aspect of the forearm, but for the most part patients do not emphasize this aspect. Although there is no functional limitation at the donor arm, strength and extension can be objectively reduced after transection of the triceps head. Another disadvantage is the limited width of the flap, so that another donor site should be considered if a broad flap is needed. As a solution to this problem, Katsaros suggested dividing a long flap and positioning both skin islands adjacent to each other, so that the flap width is doubled and the donor site still can be closed directly [180]. Another possibility to overcome this problem is pre-transfer skin expansion [351], but this technique cannot be performed in patients with malignant tumors needing primary reconstruction.

Flap Raising

Patient Positioning

The upper arm is disinfected completely from the shoulder and axilla down to the distal forearm and brought in an abducted and supine position. In the elbow, the arm is moderately flexed. In this position, flap raising can be carried out simultaneously with tumor resection in the head and neck area. No specific preoperative measures are necessary for elevating the lateral arm flap, and there is no need to use a tourniquet.

Standard Flap Design

For most indications, the flap dimensions vary between 7 and 12 cm in length and 5 and 6 cm in width. The central axis of the skin island lies over the septum between the brachialis and triceps muscle (lateral intermuscular septum), which is represented by the interconnection of the lateral epicondyle and the insertion of the deltoid muscle. The skin paddle covers the biceps and brachialis muscle anterior and the lateral head of the triceps muscle posterior to the septum, with a maximum width of 7 cm. The distal pole of the flap is outlined 1–2 cm proximal to the epicondyle, and the proximal pole is placed 4–6 cm below the deltoid insertion. An incision is made for exposure of the proximal vascular pedicle.

Step 1 At the posterior circumference of the flap, the skin incision is made perpendicularly through the subcutaneous fatty tissue until the brachial fascia is reached. During the entire flap raising procedure, the skin paddle should not be separated from the underlying fascia, which forms the intermuscular septum and thus contains the septocutaneous flap vessels.

Step 2 After identifying the fascia, it is incised at the posterior periphery of the flap, and the lateral head of the triceps muscle is exposed. By careful elevation of the fascia, the dissection proceeds bluntly in an anterior direction until the lateral intermuscular septum is reached. This septum separates the triceps from the brachialis muscle. On the surface of the septum, the septocutaneous perforating vessels from the posterior radial collateral artery (PRCA) become visible.

Step 3 Flap raising is continued at the anterior margin of the flap, where the brachial fascia is identified and than incised. In the subfascial plane, the flap is now undermined until the anterior aspect of the lateral intermuscular septum has been reached. The brachioradialis muscle, which partly originates from the distal part of the septum, and the brachialis muscle are exposed. In addition to the septocutaneous perforators, which also become visible at the anterior aspect of the septum, the fascia contains the posterior cutaneous nerve of the forearm (PCNF). This branch of the radial nerve provides sensation distal to the lateral epicondyle at the forearm and is sacrificed during flap raising.

Step 4 In the close-up view, three perforating vessels can be seen arising from the base of the intermuscular septum to the skin. The PRCA, from which the perforators branch off, runs along the base of the septum distally where it anastomoses with the interosseous recurrent artery. It is accompanied by the PCNF, which later is transected at the point where the artery enters the proximal pole of the flap. The base of the septum is still firmly attached to the humerus bone.

Step 5 Before the septum is incised distally, the strong radial nerve is palpated anterior to the septum between the brachioradialis and brachialis muscle. The nerve is exposed at the distal third of the upper arm by careful and blunt separation of the muscle fibers. The nerve is accompanied by the anterior radial collateral artery, which does not contribute to flap perfusion. After identifying the nerve, it can easily be protected during the following separation of the lateral intermuscular septum from the humerus bone.

Step 6 The intermuscular septum is perpendicularly incised at the distal flap pole to the level of the periosteum. The flap is elevated, and the base of the septum becomes visible. Here, the PRCA and the PCNF are transected and ligated at the distal end of the septum directly over the periosteum of the humerus bone.

25

Now the base of the intermuscular septum, which contains the PRCA, is separated from the humerus. Care must be taken not to miss the pedicle, which runs close to the bone. Therefore, it is recommended to perform the dissection directly at the periosteum. With direct visualization of the radial nerve, this is possible with no risk of injury to either the radial nerve or the vascular pedicle. Having the scissors always in contact with the periosteum guarantees maintaining the right dissection plane.

Flap elevation is continued in the cranial direction, where the vascular pedicle is still covered by the bellies of the brachialis and triceps muscle. Before the dissection of the pedicle is continued, the PCNA is revealed, which branches off from the radial nerve to enter the septum and ramify in the subcutaneous tissue of the flap. Together with the PRCA, this cutaneous nerve represents the neurovascular pedicle of the flap.

In the close-up view of the neurovascular hilum, it can be seen that the radial nerve, the PCNA, and the vascular pedicle run quite closely together, so that proximal dissection of the pedicle must now be performed with great care to prevent any injury to the radial nerve.

For further exposure of the pedicle, the septum is transected at the superior pole of the flap while the neurovascular pedicle is carefully protected. The flap is now completely elevated, and the PRCA, which is always accompanied by two veins, is traced in the proximal direction along the spiral groove of the humerus.

To lengthen the pedicle up to the brachial artery, the dissection can be extended proximally between the lateral and long heads of the triceps muscle. To this end, these muscles have to be split to reach the takeoff of the profunda brachii artery from the brachial artery. Using this technique, it is important to preserve the branches of the radial nerve to the triceps muscle. If the standard pedicle length of 6–8 cm is sufficient, the dissection ends where the fibers of the lateral head of the triceps limit further exposure of the profunda brachii artery along the spiral groove. At the proximal end of the pedicle, the comitant veins are bluntly separated from the artery. The PCNA always has to be transected at the cranial flap pole and can be used for neurocutaneous reinnervation. Direct wound closure can be accomplished if the width of the flap does not exceed 6–7 cm.

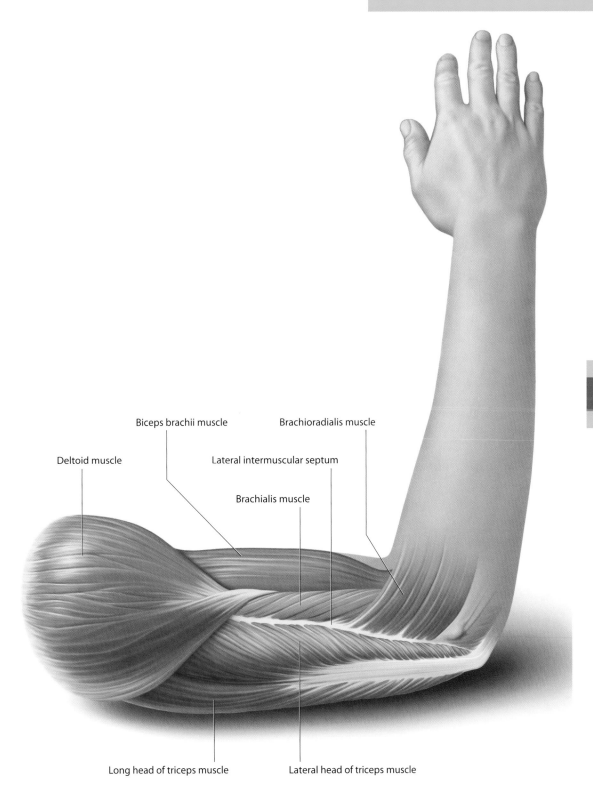

Deltoid muscle

Biceps brachii muscle

Brachioradialis muscle

Lateral intermuscular septum

Brachialis muscle

Long head of triceps muscle

Lateral head of triceps muscle

Muscles of the upper arm

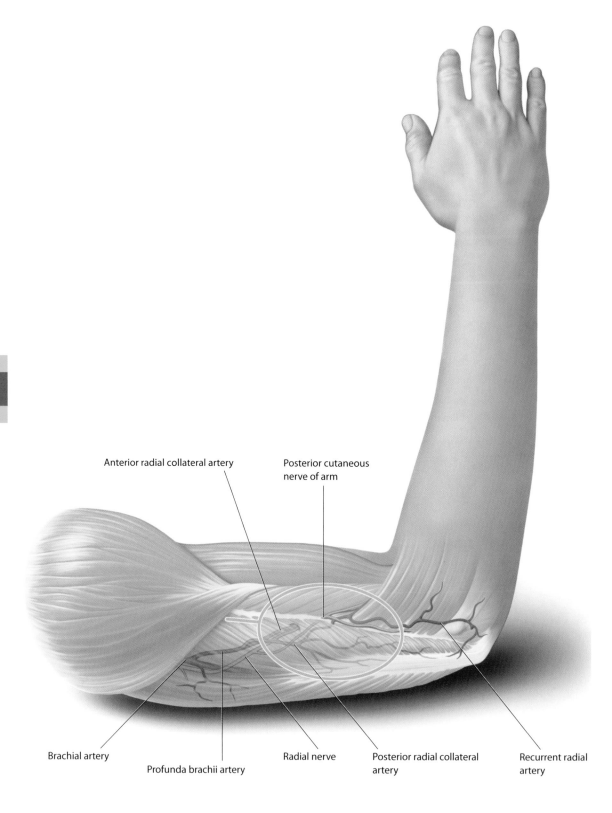

Anterior radial collateral artery

Posterior cutaneous
nerve of arm

Brachial artery

Profunda brachii artery

Radial nerve

Posterior radial collateral
artery

Recurrent radial
artery

Vascular system and standard design of the lateral upper arm flap

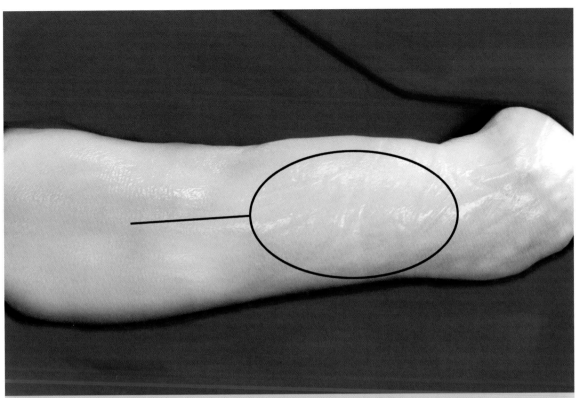

Position of standard skin paddle

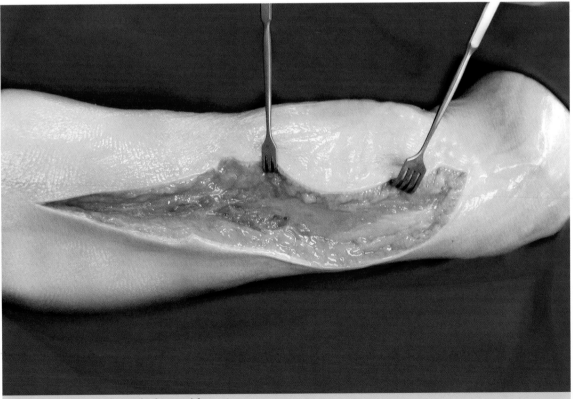

Step 1 • Incision through skin and fatty tissue

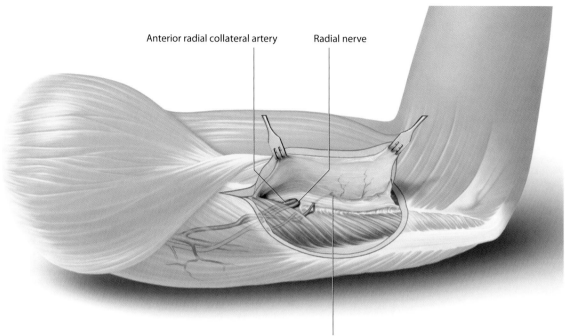

Anterior radial collateral artery   Radial nerve

Posterior radial collateral artery and septocutaneous perforators

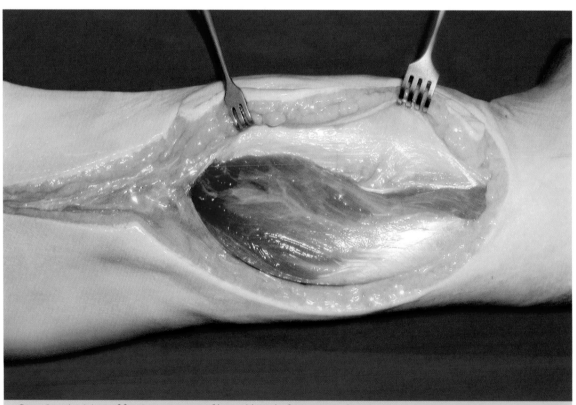

Step 2 • Incision of fascia, exposure of lateral head of triceps and septum

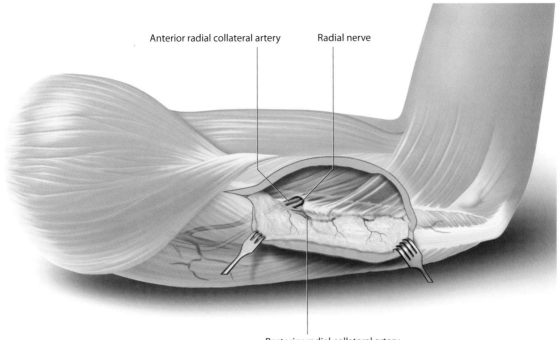

Anterior radial collateral artery   Radial nerve

Posterior radial collateral artery

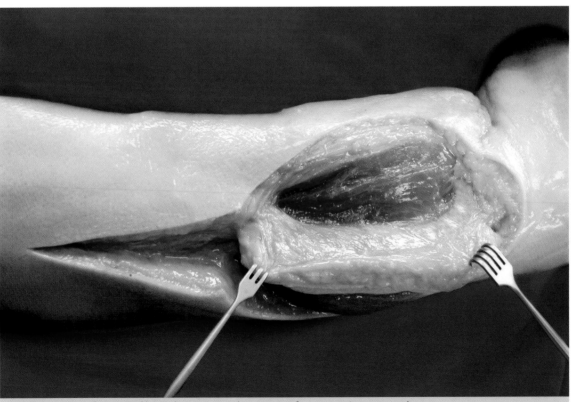

Step 3 • Identification of lateral intermuscular septum from anterior approach

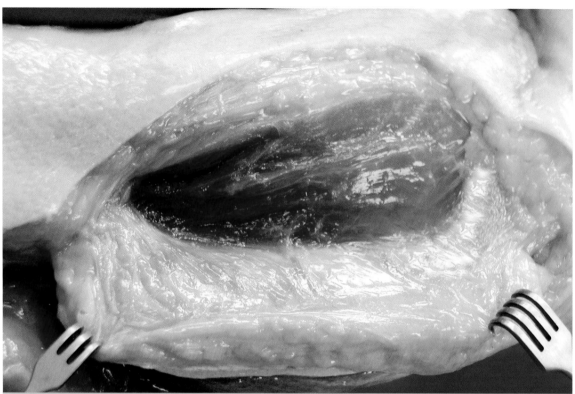

Step 4 • Identification of septocutaneous perforators

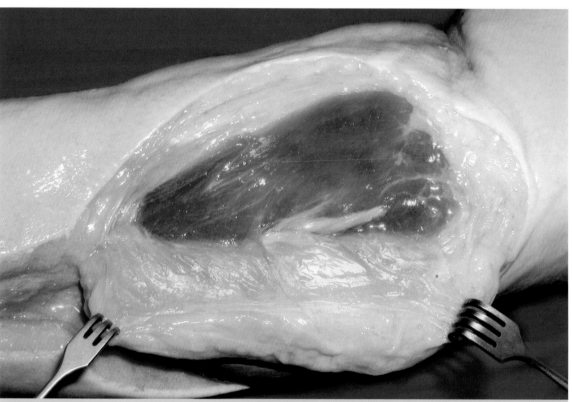

Step 5 • Exposure of radial nerve

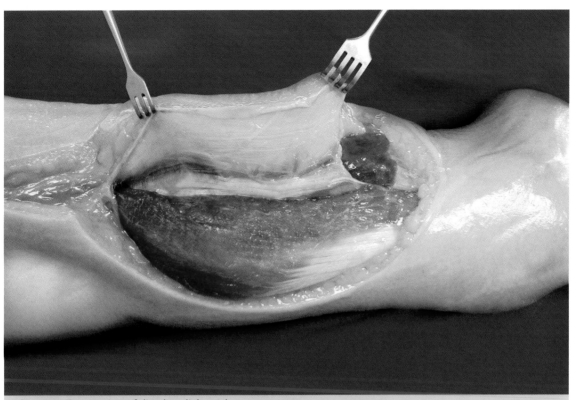

Step 6 • Transection of distal pedicle and septum

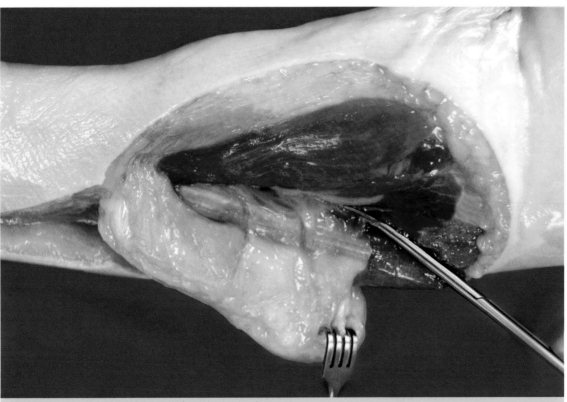

Step 7 • Detachment of septum from humerus bone

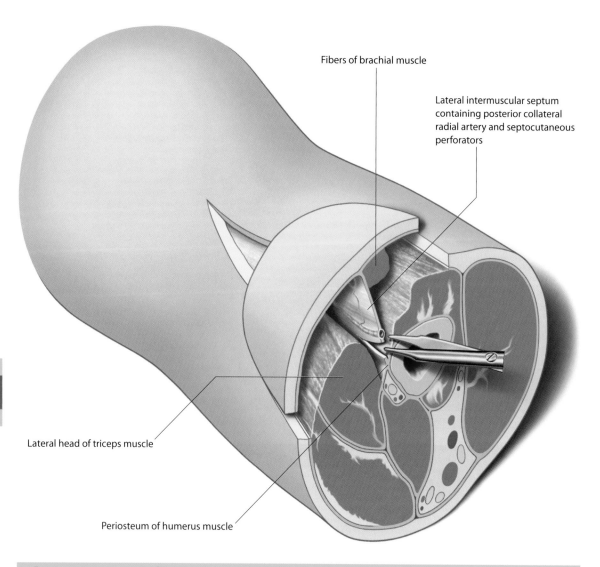

Fibers of brachial muscle

Lateral intermuscular septum containing posterior collateral radial artery and septocutaneous perforators

Lateral head of triceps muscle

Periosteum of humerus muscle

34

Cross-section anatomy of the right arm, epiperiosteal detachment of lateral intermuscular septum

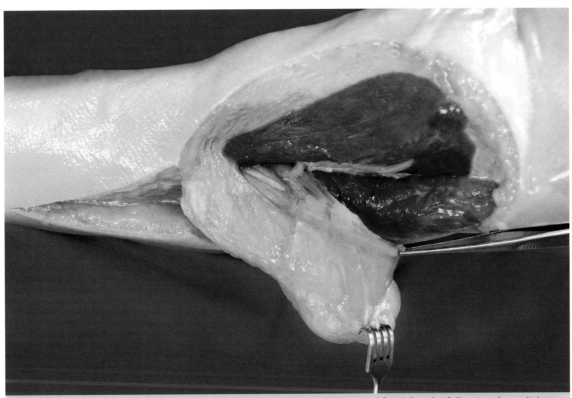

Step 8 • Identification of posterior cutaneous nerve of the arm (PCNA) and flap hilum by following the radial nerve

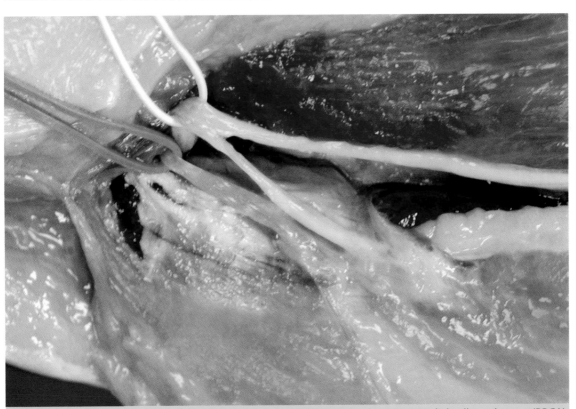

Step 9 • Separating the PCNA, branching off from the radial nerve and posterior radial collateral artery (PRCA)

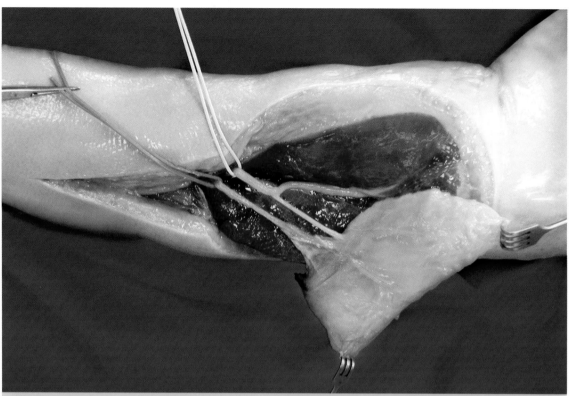

Step 10 • Further exposure of the pedicle

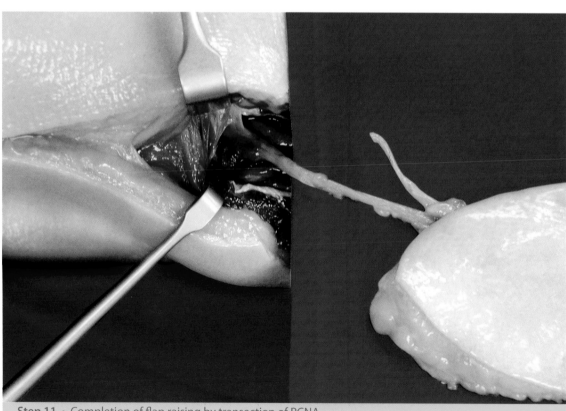

Step 11 • Completion of flap raising by transection of PCNA

Comments

Planning

The muscle groove between the brachialis and biceps brachii muscle might be mistaken for the lateral intermuscular septum. Check the position of the brachialis muscle by palpation. The skin island should not be too narrow, because the intermuscular septum can easily be missed.

Steps 1, 3: The intermuscular septum should not be injured by undermining the skin paddle. The incision down to the fascia should be made perpendicularly through the fatty tissue. Incise the fascia until the muscle fibers become clearly visible.

Step 2: The intermuscular septum can easily be injured in sharp instead of blunt dissection.

Step 6: The septum must be detached from the bone at the level of the periosteum. Control the correct plane of dissection by direct palpation of the humerus bone.

Step 7: The vascular pedicle might be missed if the septum is not incised directly at the humerus. Keep the scissor in direct contact with the periosteum while transecting the septum.

Steps 9, 10: The vascular pedicle can easily be injured as it enters the flap at its cranial pole. Separate the pedicle from the radial nerve carefully and place a loop around the vessels before the cranial pole of the flap is completely circumcised.

Anterolateral Thigh/ Vastus Lateralis Flap

39

Wolff/Hölzle, *Raising of Microvascular Flaps 2nd ed.*,
DOI: 10.1007/978-3-642-13831-7_3, © Springer-Verlag Berlin Heidelberg 2011

Development and Indications

In 1984, Song and co-workers described the thigh as a donor site for three new flaps, which they raised from its posterior, anteromedial, and antero-lateral aspects [361]. Of these three flaps, the anterolateral thigh flap became most popular, especially in head and neck reconstruction. Although originally described as a fasciocutaneous flap that is fed by a septocutaneous perforator of the descending branch of the lateral circumflex femoral artery, the design of the flap significantly depends on the course and location of the cutaneous vessels, the anatomy of which can vary considerably. Because the perforator often takes its course through the vastus lateralis muscle instead of running strictly along the intermuscular septum, parts of the vastus lateralis muscle have to be included in the flap in these cases. In addition to the possibility of raising large skin paddles on a single perforating vessel, the vastus lateralis muscle can be transferred as a muscle-only flap, since it is safely perfused by the descending branch. Thus, a number of flap raising possibilities exist at the anterolateral thigh, offering a wide spectrum of flaps to be harvested. In one of the first large clinical series, Zhou et al. described successful transplantation of this flap in 32 patients, most of them having defects in the region of the face and scalp [450]. Based on a single perforator, a flap design was described extending in length from the distal end of the tensor fasciae latae muscle to 7 cm above the patella and in width from the medial edge of the rectus femoris muscle to the lateral intermuscular septum. According to Koshima and co-workers, who reported on 22 reconstructions of head and neck defects, the flaps can be up to 25 cm in length and 18 cm in width [202]. Two years later, the same author combined the anterolateral thigh flap with neighboring skin, myocutaneous, and bone flaps using the lateral circumflex femoral system to treat massive composite defects of the head and neck, performing an additional anastomosis at the distal end of the descending branch [209]. In 1995, the usefulness of the anterolateral thigh flap to cover defects in the lower extremity was demonstrated by Pribaz and co-workers, especially because of the possibility of harvesting and transferring the flap under epidural anesthesia [297]. An important variation of designing the anterolateral thigh flap was introduced by Kimura et al. in 1996, who performed a primary radical thinning procedure, only leaving a small cuff of fatty tissue along the perforator [194]. With this procedure, ultra-thin flaps could be created, which are very useful for covering superficial skin defects [57, 194, 419, 441]. To improve intraoral defect cover, Wolff et al. also performed de-epithelialization of the thinned flaps to create a mucosa-like flap surface [432]. In the following years, the exceptionally wide spectrum of indications and the high reliability of the flap was reported, especially from authors from the Asian countries. In 2002, Wei et al. published a series of 672 anterolateral thigh flaps with total flap failure in only 12 patients [419]. An even larger number of 1284 patients was presented by Gedebou and Wei in the same year, who described the anterolateral thigh flap as one of the most useful soft tissue flaps, especially in head and neck reconstruction [117].The vastus lateralis muscle was first used as a pedicled regional flap to treat trochanteric pressure sores [45, 94, 145, 263] and to repair defects at the gluteal region [1] and knee [371]. In 1987, Drimmer and Krasna described myocutaneous vastus lateralis flaps in four patients to treat decubitus at the gluteal region [96]; later, Rojviroy et al. used this pedicled myocutaneous flap to cover trochanteric pressure in paraplegic patients [313]. The first microsurgical transfer of the vastus lateralis muscle flap to the oral cavity was reported by Wolff in 1992 [424], who covered intraoral defects using myofascial and myocutaneous flaps. In further clinical series, the same author described the usefulness of the muscle in combination with one or more skin paddles for reconstruction in the head and neck including the skull base and perforating defects of the cheek [422, 423, 426, 432]. Because the muscle flap can be raised independently of the cutaneous vessels, flat and fascial covered flaps can be created from the distal half of the vastus lateralis, making it possible to obtain vascular pedicles up to 15 cm long.

Anatomy

The vastus lateralis is the largest portion of the quadriceps femoris muscle and is located between the vastus intermedius, biceps, and rectus femoris muscle. It originates from the intertrochanteric line, the greater trochanter, gluteal tuberosity, and the lateral intermuscular septum. Together with the other muscles of the quadriceps group, its tendon builds the patellar ligament and thus is a strong extensor of the leg [314, 420]. Together with the gluteus maximus muscle, the vastus lateralis forms the vastogluteal muscle sling, leading to an extension, external rotation, and adduction of the leg [410]. The muscle, measuring approximately 10×25cm, is innervated by a motor branch of the femoral nerve. This nerve enters the muscle at its medial border in the proximal and interomedial segments and follows the course of the main dominant vascular pedicle. The vascular supply of the vastus lateralis muscle comes from the descending branch of the lateral circumflex femoral artery and its two venae comitantes, with a diameter of 1.5–2.5 mm (artery) and 1.8–3.3 mm (veins) [424]. According to Mathes and Nahai, the muscle has a type I pattern of circulation, providing perfusion of the entire muscle from this dominant vascular pedicle [245, 246]. Additional minor pedicles reach the muscle far proximally (transverse branch of the lateral circumflex femoral artery) and distally (lateral superior genicular artery), with no significance for microvascular transfer. After it arises from the lateral circumflex femoral artery, the descending branch reaches the medial rim of the vastus lateralis muscle in its proximal segment and courses distally to communicate with the superior genicular artery. Because the entire muscle is supplied by side branches of the artery, muscle flaps can be raised from each portion of the vastus lateralis. The vascular pedicle can easily be exposed in the triangle that is built by the tensor fasciae latae, vastus lateralis, and rectus femoris muscle in the proximal third of the thigh. Here, the pedicle has a length of 6–8 cm before entering the vastus lateralis muscle. When used as a rotation flap, the proximally based muscle can reach the trochanteric, gluteal, perineal, and lower abdominal regions. As a distally based flap, the lower third of the muscle, which is supplied by the distal minor pedicle, can be used for defect cover around the knee [371]. Apart from the blood supply to the vastus lateralis muscle, the descending branch divides into the myo- or septocutaneous branches, giving the anatomical basis of the myocutaneous vastus lateralis or septocutaneous anterolateral thigh flap. These flaps, which can be considered as one entity, only differ in the amount of muscle tissue that is included during flap raising. Depending on the course of the cutaneous vessels, a portion of the medial edge of the vastus lateralis muscle has to be removed, forming a protective cuff around the myocutaneously running vessels. According to the results of anatomical investigations, the dominant cutaneous vessel of the anterolateral thigh was found to have a myocutaneous course in 80–90% of individuals. However, since the myocutaneous vessel traverses the muscle close to its medial edge, a small cuff of muscle must be included, but the function of the vastus lateralis can be preserved completely. For extended and deep defects, larger portions of the vastus lateralis muscle, the same size as the skin paddle, can be harvested, so that voluminous myocutaneous vastus lateralis flaps are created. In only 10–20% of patients does the dominant cutaneous vessel have a direct course to the skin, running along the septum between the rectus femoris and vastus lateralis muscle and piercing the fascia lata without traversing the vastus lateralis muscle. These anterolateral thigh flaps are raised without any muscle tissue and thus provide thin and pliable skin paddles, well suited for reconstructions in the head and neck area, including the oral cavity. In a number of anatomical investigations and clinical series, the vascular anatomy of the anterolateral thigh was found to vary; therefore the cutaneous vessel must always be exposed before the location of the skin paddle can be determined precisely. The dominant cutaneous vessel can be found within a 4-cm radius at the midpoint of a line between the anterior superior iliac spine and the lateral border of the patella in nearly all cases [245, 424]. To facilitate exposure of the cutaneous perforator, preoperative mapping using audible Doppler is generally recommended. Although the exact course of this dominant cutaneous vessel can only be explored during flap raising, a myocutaneous pattern can be expected if the Doppler signal is detected not directly over the palpable groove between the rectus and vastus lateralis muscle, but 2–4 cm lateral to the septum above the medial portion of the muscle. Once the exact location of the perforator is defined, the skin paddle can be outlined over the middle third of the lateral thigh between the medial border of the rectus femoris and the lateral border of the vastus lateralis muscle, up to 12×30 cm [245]. Depending on the exact location of the main cutaneous perforator, the length of the vascular pedicle varies, being 12 cm on average [354]. Apart from this main perforator, the descending branch provides one to three additional cutaneous branches, reaching the skin more distally to the main perforator. Whereas the most distally located of these additional vessels are not reliable for skin perfusion, a second perforator can be found in about 90% of all cases 4–9 cm distal to the main perforator, making it possible to build a second independent skin paddle. Like the dominant perforator, this additional cutaneous vessel has a myocutaneous course in 80–90% of patients, piercing the muscle 2–5 cm from its medial rim. The variations of the course of the cutaneous perforators were described in detail by Sieh, who found vertical musculocutaneous perforators in 57% of patients and horizontal myocutaneous perforators in 27%, whereas vertical septocutaneous perforators were only found in 11% and horizontal septocutaneous perforators in 5% of their 36 clinical cases [354]. The length of the cutaneous perforating vessels varied between 3.6 and 7.7 cm.

Sensory innervation of the perforator flap skin paddle can be established by anastomosing branches of the lateral cutaneous femoral nerve [424]. In an anatomical and clinical study, Ribuffo et al. described that a superior nerve branch innervates 25%, whereas a medial branch innervates 60% of the vascular territory, so that a selection can be made according to the location and size of the skin paddle without sacrificing the whole lateral cutaneous femoral nerve [306]. The vascular anatomy of the cutaneous perforators of the lateral thigh was found to give a suitable basis for primary flap-thinning procedures, which were first described by Kimura and Satoh in 1996 [194]. In their first five cases, they removed the subcutaneous fatty tissue uniformly from the whole flap except for the region around the perforator, obtaining a flap thickness of only 3–4 mm. Further experience with primary thinning has shown that the radical removal of fatty tissue does not impair flap perfusion if the subdermal vascular plexus is preserved and attention is paid to the vascular territory of the corresponding flap vessels [203]. Although Ross and coworkers found a higher complication rate in their clinical series [315] and Alkureishi et al. experimentally found reduced dye perfusion of the thinned flaps [5], the literature generally reports low complication rates [5, 203, 419, 432]. All authors agree, however, that flap thinning must be performed with a high degree of technical skill and exact knowledge of the vascular anatomy. A prerequisite for successful thinning is the preservation of the subdermal vascular plexus, which means that the minimal flap thickness should not be less than 3–4 mm. Under these conditions, the size of the vascular territory of a thinned flap corresponds to conventional flaps [203, 275, 419]. Whereas Kimura et al. (1996) emphasized that the vessel anatomy of the anterolateral thigh flap is especially well suited for flap thinning [194] if the perforator courses directly to the skin, other authors performed additional dissection through the vastus lateralis muscle in the case of a myocutaneous vessel course to obtain thinned flaps [49, 117, 419, 432]. Using this technique, it is possible to raise voluminous, extensive flaps as well as very thin small flaps from the same donor region.

Advantages and Disadvantages

Since its first description by Song in 1984 [361], the anterolateral thigh has been developed as one of the most preferred donor sites for soft tissue reconstruction, especially in the head and neck area. With a failure rate of

43

less than 2%, Wei and co-workers performed reconstruction in 660 cases, most of them with defects in the head and neck region. Irrespective of whether the skin vessels were septo- or myocutaneous, they were able to raise versatile soft tissue flaps in which thickness and volume could be adjusted to cover the full extent of the defect [419]. According to their experience, the anterolateral thigh could replace most other donor sites for soft tissue free flaps. In addition to the exceptional and promising experience of Wei's group, similar results have been reported by a number of other authors, describing success rates of approximately 95% with a wide indicational spectrum, reaching from perforator-based ultrathin skin flaps to myocutaneous vastus lateralis and extensive chimeric flaps, which include parts of the surrounding muscles and even segments of the iliac crest [209]. The donor site can be closed primarily if the width of the flap does not exceed approximately 8 cm, and there are no significant functional or aesthetic impairments at the thigh even after harvesting a large portion of the vastus lateralis muscle. However, when raising flaps from the anterolateral thigh, the surgeon must be aware of possible variations in vascular anatomy. Besides the variability of the course and location of the main cutaneous perforator, the absence of any cutaneous branches is possible in rare cases [202, 215, 419, 422] and has been described to occur in up to 5.4% of patients [190]. Although the branching pattern of the skin vessels in a series of 74 clinical cases was classified into eight categories, no variation was found that made flap raising impossible. In this series, 2.3 perforators per case were found, 82% of them with a myocutaneous course, branching off at different levels from the descending branch, the lateral circumflex femoral artery, the transverse branch, or directly from the profunda femoris artery [13, 190]. Because the veins that accompany the nutrient artery can show different back-flow strength, venous return should be checked before anastomosis. In a clinical study of 115 flap raising procedures at the anterolateral thigh, the descending branch was found to be absent in 22.6%, replaced by the medial descending branch or other strong muscle branches [13]. Although in this study the anatomical course of the descending branch was classified into six different categories, flap elevation was possible in all cases, because at least one cutaneous perforator was always observed. For intraoral defect cover, the thickness of the flap can be disadvantageous, especially in myocutaneous flaps carrying a large portion of muscle tissue. In these cases, muscle or fatty tissue has to be primarily removed without injuring the cutaneous vessel, but these thinning procedures should only be carried out by experienced surgeons with precise knowledge of the vascular anatomy. Because of neurogenic muscle atrophy and secondary shrinkage, purely muscular flaps only have a limited indication for intraoral soft tissue replacement [427]. The width of the skin paddle in myocutaneous flaps is limited to about 8–10 cm; in males, substantial hair growth can sometimes be observed at the lateral thigh. Apart from some loss of sensation, donor site morbidity is low but can increase when wider flaps needing a split-thickness skin graft for closure of the donor site or flaps including significant parts of the vastus lateralis muscle have been harvested [192].

Flap Raising

Preoperative Management

Despite the anatomical variations described for the vascular pedicle of the anterolateral thigh/vastus lateralis flap, angiography is not helpful in locating the variable positions of the septo- or myocutaneous branches of the descending artery. Preoperative evaluation of the perforators should be performed using a Doppler probe by carefully auscultating the skin in the region of the intermuscular septum and over the medial parts of the vastus lateralis muscle.

Patient Positioning

The patient is placed in a supine position, and the entire leg is included in the operating field to allow for free positioning of the extremity and for modifying the flap design if necessary. Circular disinfection is performed from the hip down to the lower leg.

Flap Design

The standard skin paddle of the flap may be extended from the rectus femoris to the tensor fasciae latae or biceps femoris muscle, covering the middle third of the thigh. The center of the flap depends on the individual location of the perforator(s), which can be found a few centimeters proximal to the midpoint of the interconnection between the anterior superior iliac spine and the patella in most patients. Because of the variability of the perforators, the skin paddle is not peritomized until the perforator is identified from the medial border of the flap. The incision to expose the vascular pedicle is marked between the tensor and rectus femoris muscle at the proximal thigh.

Step 1 The incision is made over the rectus femoris muscle, maintaining a safe distance from the intermuscular septum, which can be palpated between the rectus and vastus lateralis muscle. The location of the septum is represented by the interconnecting line between the anterior superior iliac spine and the lateral border of the patella. Cranially, the incision is extended along the palpable groove between the rectus femoris and tensor muscle for exposure of the vascular pedicle. The fascia lata still remains intact. It should again be mentioned that before the skin paddle is outlined, the perforator(s) must be visualized in the subfascial plane to determine the center of the flap.

Step 2 The fascia is incised along the rectus femoris muscle so that the intermuscular septum is completely included in the flap. To gain optimal access to the pedicle, the proximal incision is placed along the groove between the tensor and the rectus muscle.

The rectus femoris and tensor muscles are bluntly separated from each other, and by retracting the rectus femoris muscle medially, the vascular pedicle becomes visible. At the middle third of the thigh where the skin perforators are expected to be, the intermuscular septum is left intact.

Step 3

A vessel loop is placed around the pedicle, and the intermuscular septum is opened with scissors directly at the lateral rim of the rectus muscle. Great care must be taken not to transect perforating vessels arising from the descending branch into the septum. The use of magnifying glasses is recommended to identify the perforators more easily.

Step 4

It can clearly be seen that the pedicle consists of one artery, the descending branch, two comitant veins, and a motor branch of the femoral nerve, innervating the vastus lateralis muscle. The pedicle runs distally underneath the anterior border of the vastus lateralis muscle to anastomose with the vascular network around the knee.

Step 5

If no septocutaneous perforators are found, myocutaneous perforators that pierce the vastus muscle along its anterior border will be present. This is the case in the majority of patients. Using magnifying glasses, these myocutaneous perforators become visible entering the muscle along its undersurface at the anterior muscle rim. Because the perforators traverse the muscle closely underneath its surface, their pulsation can often be observed and the tiny vessels can be followed to the skin paddle. In this cadaver, three myocutaneous perforators are seen penetrating the vastus lateralis muscle at its anterior border and entering the skin paddle, which now can be designated. Distally, the vascular pedicle is exposed above the intermedius fascia and than ligated.

Step 6

After identification of the perforators, the skin island is peritomized completely, including the deep fascia, and fixated at the anterior border of the muscle to prevent shearing of the perforators. Again it must be emphasized that final determination of the flap margins is only possible after the perforators have been visualized.

Step 7

By retracting the rectus femoris muscle, the vascular pedicle is followed distally and exposed on the surface of the vastus intermedius muscle. With careful elevation of the anterior rim of the vastus lateralis, a number of vascular branches become visible, reaching the muscle and the skin paddle.

Step 8

Although the myocutaneous perforators run through the muscle for only a few centimeters, a large segment of the vastus muscle is included to ensure that all perforating branches are included. Starting distally, the muscle is dissected in the plane above the intermedius fascia, until the anterior rim of the vastus lateralis is nearly reached. Even though the pedicle is already ligated distally, additional muscle branches will be transected during dissection of the muscle segment, which then have to be cauterized or clipped.

Step 9

Step 10   The neurovascular pedicle is now isolated from the surrounding muscles proximal to the flap, carefully leaving the fascia, which forms the intermuscular septum and maintains the perforating vessels intact. Further muscular branches to the intermedius muscle, which can mostly be found in the proximal part of the pedicle, must be ligated.

Step 11   Flap raising is finished by further dissection of the vascular pedicle in the proximal direction, until the lateral circumflex femoral artery is reached. At the cranial pole of the flap, residual fibers of the vastus lateralis are transected, protecting the pedicle to free the myocutaneous paddle completely.

Step 12   The components of the neurovascular pedicle are bluntly separated from each other, and the flap is now ready for microvascular transplantation. It can be seen that the flap vessels branch off from the lateral circumflex femoral artery. Direct closure is possible if the width of the skin paddle does not exceed 8–9 cm. The Burow triangles must be excised at the cranial and caudal flap poles to prevent dog-ear formation following linear closure.

Myofascial Flap

Flap Design

To raise a muscle-only flap, skin, subcutaneous tissue and fascia are incised along the intermuscular septum, which is palpated between the rectus and vastus lateralis muscles.

Step 1   After subfascial exposure of the vastus lateralis muscle, dissection of the pedicle is performed proximally, elevating and retracting the rectus femoris muscle. A vessel loop is placed around the descending branch and concomitant veins.

Step 2   The vessels can now be followed easily to the distal parts of the muscle, where a myofascial flap is outlined. Since no particular care is needed for the perforating vessels, flap design is quite variable but should not exceed the borders of the vastus lateralis muscle. Nevertheless, before raising the flap, the vascular branches to the muscle segment intended to be elevated must clearly be identified.

Step 3   A number of side branches reach the vastus muscle from the dominant pedicle, demonstrating that almost the entire muscle can be transferred to the descending branch.

Step 4   Elevating the muscle segment at the transition of the medial to the distal third of the vastus lateralis makes it possible to obtain a long vascular pedicle, which makes this flap useful for coverage of skull base defects. As with the myocutaneous flap, a suction drain is inserted underneath the rectus muscle, and the skin is closed in layers. No immobilization of the patient is necessary.

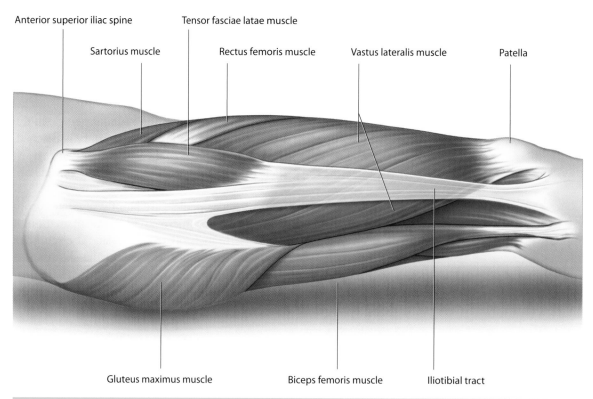

Anterior superior iliac spine

Tensor fasciae latae muscle

Sartorius muscle

Rectus femoris muscle

Vastus lateralis muscle

Patella

Gluteus maximus muscle

Biceps femoris muscle

Iliotibial tract

Muscles of the anterolateral thigh

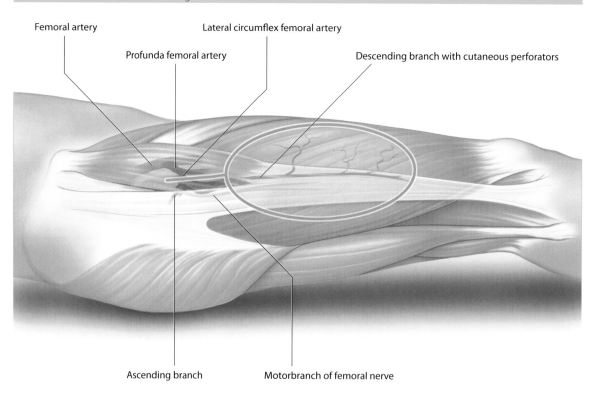

Femoral artery

Lateral circumflex femoral artery

Profunda femoral artery

Descending branch with cutaneous perforators

Ascending branch

Motorbranch of femoral nerve

Vascular system of the anterolateral thigh and standard skin paddle

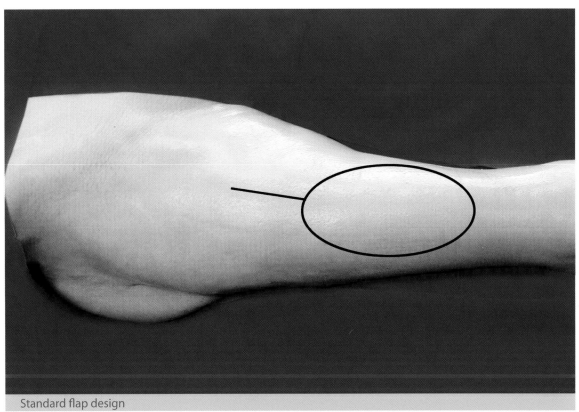

Standard flap design

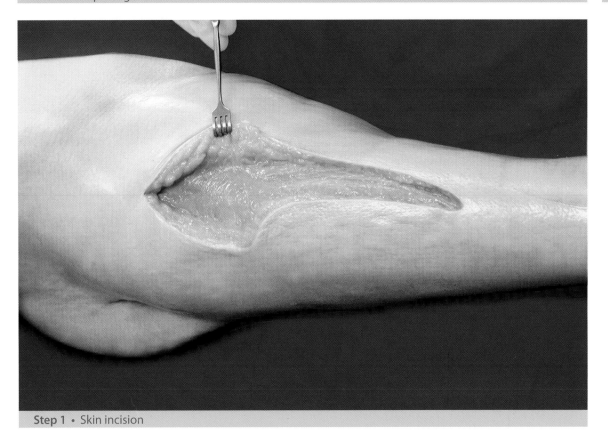

Step 1 • Skin incision

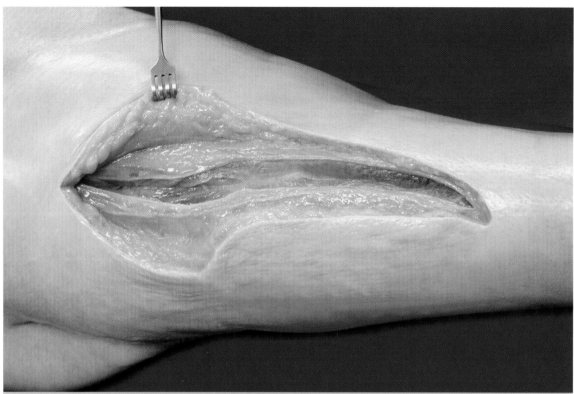

Step 2 • Incision of fascia

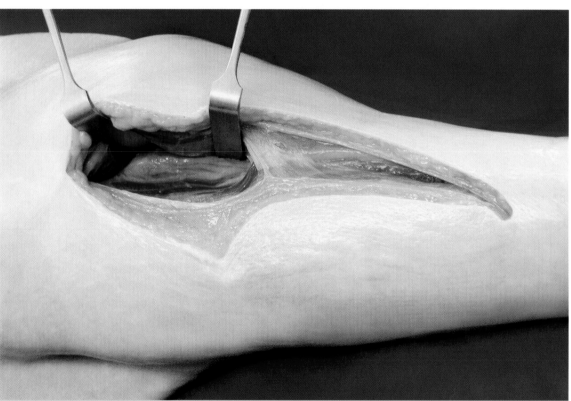

Step 3 • Exposure of vascular pedicle

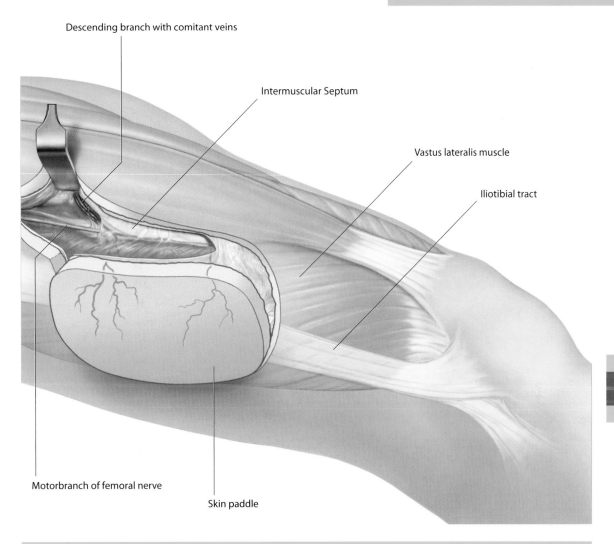

Descending branch with comitant veins

Intermuscular Septum

Vastus lateralis muscle

Iliotibial tract

Motorbranch of femoral nerve

Skin paddle

Anatomy of the intermuscular septum and course of perforators

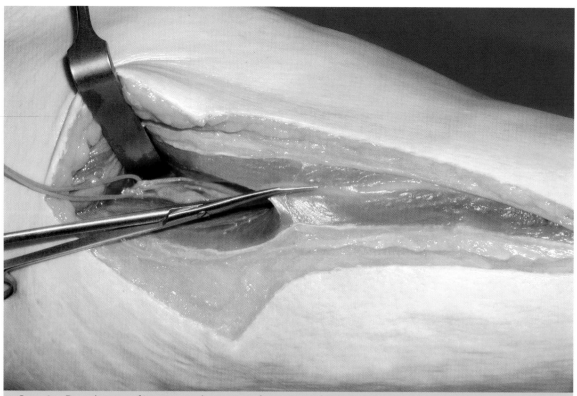

Step 4 • Detachment of intermuscular septum from rectus femoris muscle

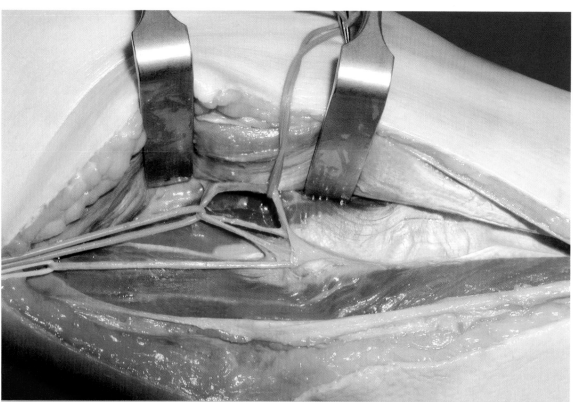

Step 5 • Separation of descending branch from concomitant veins and nerve

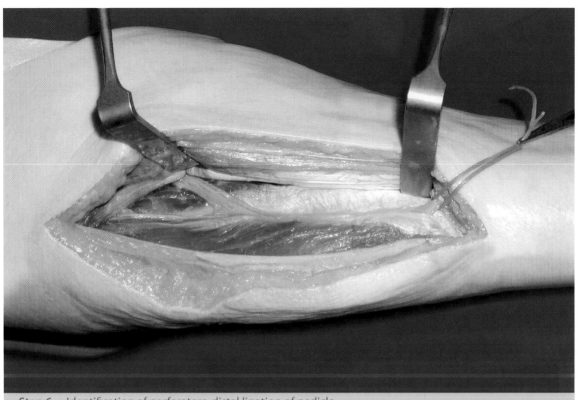

Step 6 • Identification of perforators, distal ligation of pedicle

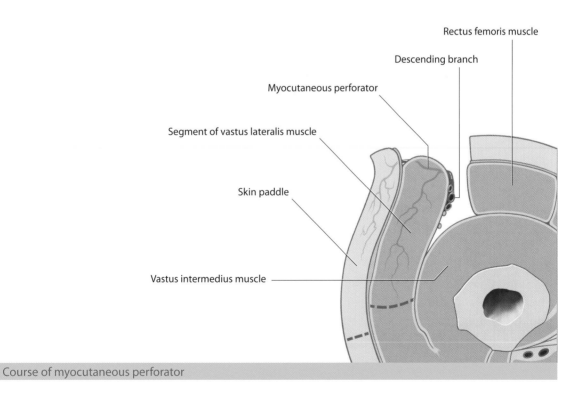

Rectus femoris muscle

Descending branch

Myocutaneous perforator

Segment of vastus lateralis muscle

Skin paddle

Vastus intermedius muscle

Course of myocutaneous perforator

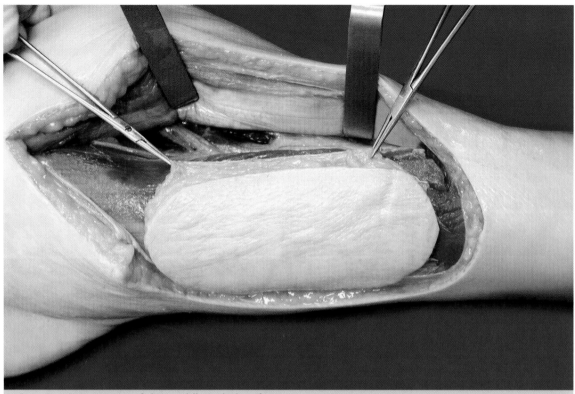

Step 7 • Circumcision of skin paddle including fascia

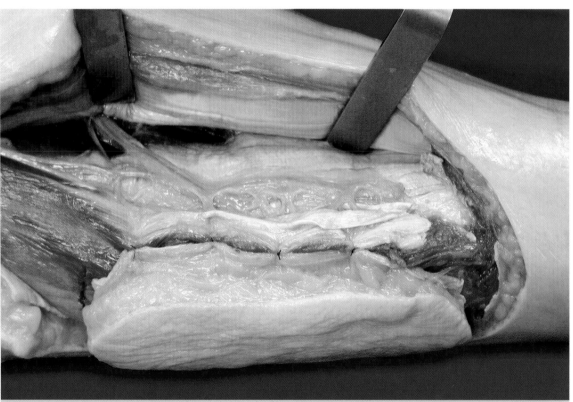

Step 8 • Fixation of skin paddle to muscle, further exposure of vascular pedicle

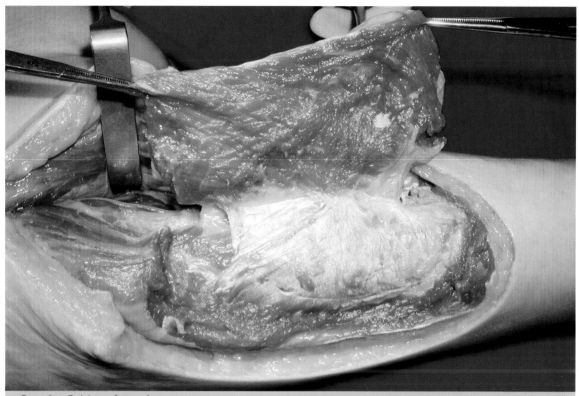

Step 9 • Raising of muscle component

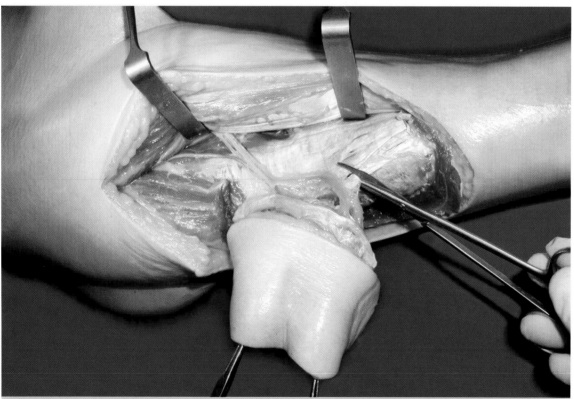

Step 10 • Dissection of vascular pedicle

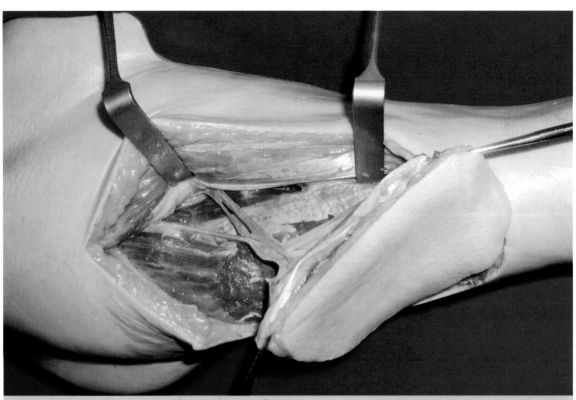

Step 11 • Complete elevation of myocutaneous flap

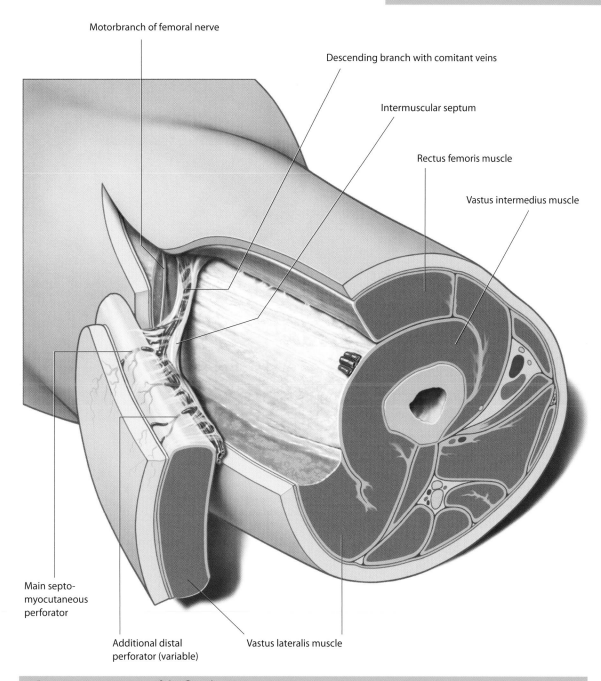

Motorbranch of femoral nerve

Descending branch with comitant veins

Intermuscular septum

Rectus femoris muscle

Vastus intermedius muscle

Main septo-
myocutaneous
perforator

Additional distal
perforator (variable)

Vastus lateralis muscle

57

Cross-section anatomy of the flap donor site

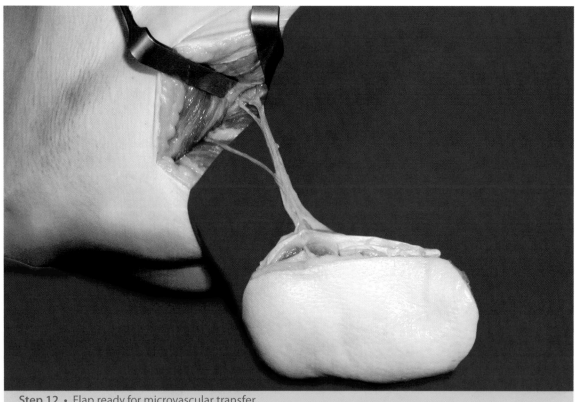

Step 12 • Flap ready for microvascular transfer

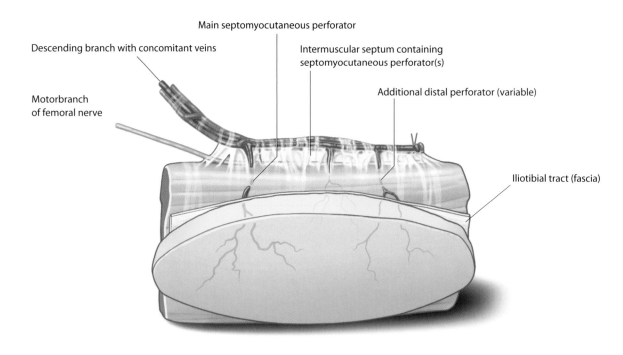

Descending branch with concomitant veins

Motorbranch
of femoral nerve

Main septomyocutaneous perforator

Intermuscular septum containing
septomyocutaneous perforator(s)

Additional distal perforator (variable)

Iliotibial tract (fascia)

Myocutaneous flap containing two perforators

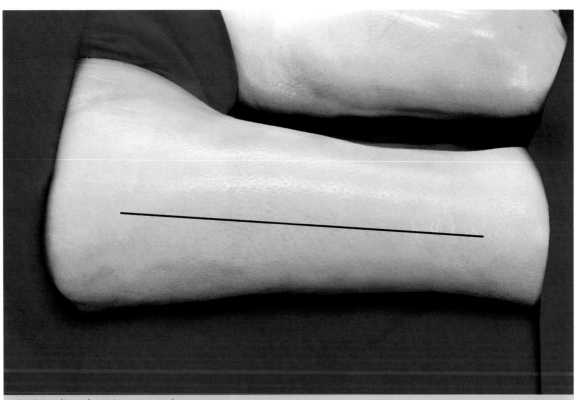

Incision line along intermuscular septum

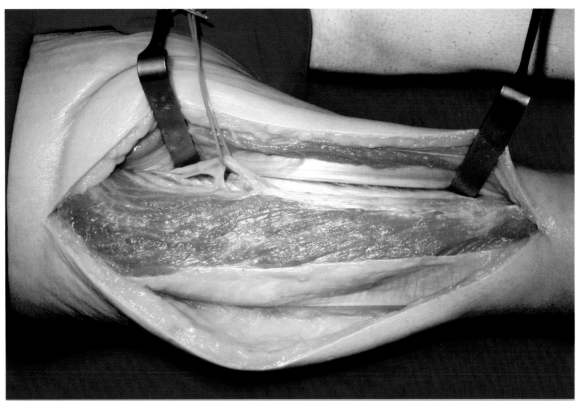

Step 1 • Proximal exposure of pedicle, incision of fascia and intermuscular septum

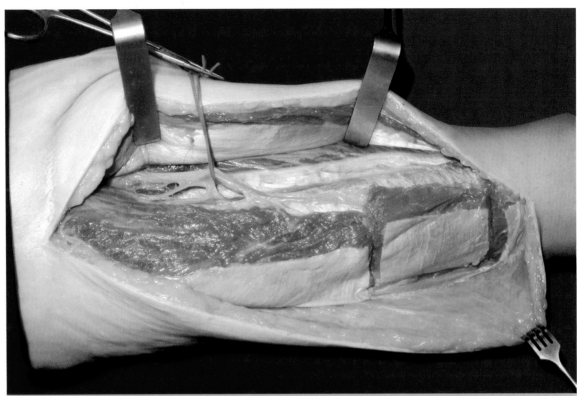

Step 2 • Defining of the muscle segment

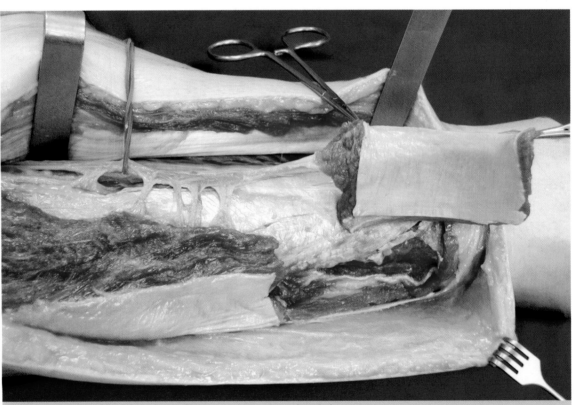

Step 3 • Elevation of the muscle segment, dissection of pedicle

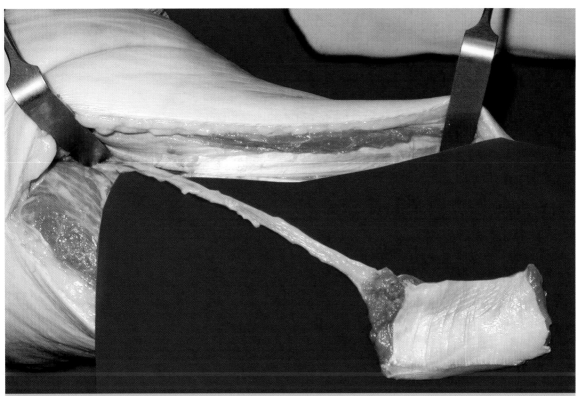

Step 4 • Myofascial vastus lateralis flap with long pedicle

Comments

Planning

The skin island should never be outlined before the main perforating vessel is exposed. The skin incision to expose the main perforating vessel should not be outlined lateral to the rectus femoris muscle, because this will injure the intermuscular septum. Preoperative mapping of the main perforator using an audible Doppler can facilitate planning of the flap design.

Step 1: If the skin incision is performed too far laterally, the cutaneous perforator will be missed or injured. If the skin incision is performed too far medially, exposure of the descending branch may become difficult. We advise that the intermuscular septum can be located preoperatively while the patient extends the leg.

Step 3: If the fascia is incised medial to the rectus femoris muscle, the descending branch cannot be exposed. Palpate the rectus femoris muscle before the fascia is opened.

Step 4: The cutaneous vessels running along the intermuscular septum can easily be injured while opening the fascia. The use of magnifying glasses may facilitate identification and preservation of the perforators running along the septum. Do not expose the cutaneous perforators in the level above the fascia to prevent shearing or stretching forces to the tiny vessels.

Step 6: The location, origin, and course of the perforators are variable. Before the skin paddle is outlined, make sure that the perforator branches off by the descending artery and pierces the fascia to enter the skin. If necessary, the transverse branch, the lateral circumflex femoral artery, or the perforator itself can serve as the vascular pedicle.

Step 9: The cutaneous vessels may be injured if the muscle cuff around the perforators is too narrow. Keep a safe three-dimensional distance around these vessels while dissecting the muscular portion of the flap.

Step 12: Blood flow can be different in both veins accompanying the descending branch. To determine the appropriate vein for anastomosis, venous return should be checked before the pedicle is completely transected.

Myofascial Flap

Steps 2, 4: Although the descending branch supplies the entire vastus lateralis muscle, perfusion of the distolateral part of the muscle can be insufficient; therefore, the muscle segment should not exceed 7–8 cm in width and should not be located at the distal quarter of the muscle.

Latissimus Dorsi Flap

Wolff/Hölzle, *Raising of Microvascular Flaps 2nd ed.*,
DOI: 10.1007/978-3-642-13831-7_4, © Springer-Verlag Berlin Heidelberg 2011

Development and Indications

Like the first myocutaneous flap, the latissimus dorsi flap was described as early as 1896 by Tansini [377] and used for defect cover following radical mastectomy by D'Este in 1912 [83]. Despite its excellent suitability for chest wall reconstruction, the flap did not become popular until the 1970s, when a number of publications appeared in which the previously described advantages were confirmed, and further indications for defect cover in the area of the shoulder and arm were proposed [43, 44, 247, 253, 260, 270, 287, 357]. The first application of a pedicled latissimus dorsi flap for reconstruction in the head and neck area was described by Quillen in 1978 [300], whereas the microvascular transfer of this flap was performed by Watson in 1979 [413]. In further publications, the reliability and safety of this flap, especially its usefulness for reconstructions in the head and neck area, was demonstrated [140, 249, 250, 307, 309, 353, 413]. In all these reports, a great variety of application possibilities were described. This broad spectrum of indications was possible because of the large amount of tissue available, offering various possibilities for changing the flap design, and the long and high-caliber vascular pedicle, making microvascular anastomoses technically easy [269, 307, 309, 312]. A particular indication of the latissimus dorsi flap is the covering of large perforating defects of the oral cavity, using two skin paddles, which can be outlined along the transverse and vertical branch of the thoracodorsal artery [18, 146, 241, 269]. The inclusion of a rib allows for an osteomyocutaneous transfer and was proposed for reconstruction of the mandible or other parts of the facial skeleton [155, 233, 240]. Another indication of this broad and flat muscle is reconstruction of the scalp, especially when used as a muscle-only flap, which is covered by a skin graft [125, 269, 312, 368], or as a myofascial flap for defect cover at the skull base [310]. Motor reinnervation of the muscle flap has been described by Harii, who connected the thoracodorsal nerve to the facial nerve for rehabilitation of the paralysed face [139]. For tongue reconstruction, an anastomosis to the hypoglossal nerve was performed [160, 309]. After de-epithelization, musculosubcutaneous flaps are obtained, which were used for contour augmentations in the head and neck area [98, 269, 309]. Apart from applications in the head and neck area, many other useful indications exist for this very popular free flap, such as reconstructions of the female breast, [44, 75, 196], chest wall, and axilla [14, 247, 253], shoulder and upper extremity, [218, 228] closure of hernias of the diaphragma [26], or other intrathoracic defects [67, 70, 352]. Moreover, defect coverages at the lower extremities [44, 84] and the sacrum [328] and treatments of chronic osteomyelitis have been performed using this flap [10, 154].

Anatomy

The latissimus dorsi is a flat, fan-like muscle that arises directly from the spinal processes of the lower six thoracic vertebrae, the lumbar and sacral vertebrae, and the dorsal iliac crest via the thoracolumbar fascia. The muscle inserts between the teres and pectoralis muscles at the humerus, and together with the teres major, it forms the posterior axillary fold. The main nutrient vessel is the thoracodorsal artery, which, like the circumflex scapular artery, arises from the subscapular artery. The vascular pedicle runs along the lateral thoracic wall at the undersurface of the latissimus muscle, regularly giving off a strong branch to the serratus anterior muscle. This serratus branch can serve as the vascular pedicle if the thoracodorsal vessels have had to be sacrificed during axillary lymph node extirpation [21, 108, 390]. The length of the extramuscular part of the vessel course varies from 6 to 16 cm, approximately 9 cm on average [21]. Apart from the aforementioned branch to the serratus muscle, on its extramuscular course, the pedicle regularly branches off to another artery to the inferior angle of scapula, mostly just proximal to the serratus branch [76]. This scapular branch courses in the fascial gliding layer between the serratus, subscapularis, and teres major muscle to the scapular bone. Thus, an isolated bone flap from the tip of the scapula, which is nourished from the vascular system of the thoracodorsal artery, can be raised, and the vascular pedicle of this inferior angle scapular bone flap is about 15 cm on average [346]. Further minor vessels branch off to the teres and subscapularis muscles. The neurovascular hilum where the pedicle enters at the undersurface of the latissimus is 1.5–3 cm away from the anterior muscle rim. At the point of origin of the subscapularis vessels, the thoracodorsal vessels have diameters of 1.5–4 mm (artery) and 3–5 mm (vein after unification of the two concomitant veins) [21]. Whereas the thoracodorsal artery mainly supplies the proximal and lateral two-thirds of the muscle, the distal parts of the latissimus dorsi are reached by perforating branches of the intercostal arteries [21]. Thus, blood supply to the flap can become tenuous when harvested from the distal and medial parts of the muscle. The intramuscular course of the thoracodorsal artery, which is directly accompanied by the thoracodorsal nerve, was investigated in detail by Tobin et al. [390] and Bartlett et al. [21]. According to their findings, shortly after entering the muscle the main vessel divides into a vertical branch, which runs parallel to the anterior border of the muscle, and a transversal branch, running parallel to the proximal muscle rim. With 94.5% [390] and 86% [21], respectively, this vascular pattern was found to be present in the vast majority of cases. This consistent vascular anatomy provides the basis for dividing the flap into two separate skin paddles and two neuromuscular units. Acryl injections into the arterial system have additionally shown that multiple secondary branches arise from the transversal and vertical branches to the surface of the muscle, forming a dense network of anastomoses [317, 318]. This network allows thinning the flap by removing the superficial muscle layers without endangering blood supply [55, 316]. Although skin paddles can be designed over any part of the muscle, blood supply can become critical at the caudal and medial parts, where only a few perforating vessels to the skin where found. The highest density of myocutaneous vessels and thus the preferable region for outlining skin paddles is parallel to the anterior or cranial borders of the muscle [21, 390]. Nevertheless, an extended skin flap up to 10 cm can be built over the distal part of the latissimus muscle, which is safely perfused by myocutaneous perforators from a proximal myocutaneous portion of the flap [146]. Because of the high density of myocutaneous perforating vessels, large skin paddles can be built along the anterior muscle border, harvesting only a narrow strip of muscle that contains the vascular pedicle [233]. Although from an anatomical point of view, flap dimensions can be extended as far as 30×40 cm [321], the ability to achieve direct wound closure limits the size of the flap; thus, depending on the patient's body shape, flap width should not exceed 10 cm [310]. In addition to this wide and safe perfusion of the latissimus muscle and overlying skin, the thoracodorsal artery contributes to the blood supply of the scapular bone, which was investigated by Coleman and Sultan [76]. According to their findings, an angular branch, nourishing the tip of the scapula, branches off from the thoracodorsal artery just proximal to the serratus branch (58%) or from the serratus branch directly (42%), allowing an osteomyocutaneous transfer of the latissimus dorsi flap. This extension of flap raising can be useful for reconstruction of the anterior mandible by giving the bone a horizontal orientation to replace the interforaminal segment [178]. There are only few variations of the vascular anatomy described in the literature, none of them affecting the possibility of raising the flap. Whereas the subscapular artery and vein arise close to each other from the axillary vessels in the majority of patients, the subscapular artery can have a distance of up to 4 cm from the vein in rare cases. Moreover, the thoracodorsal artery may arise directly from the axillary artery [21]. Satoh et al. described a rare variation of blood supply to the latissimus dorsi in a clinical case where the vascular pedicle was only rudimentarily present, so that anastomoses had to be performed on the circumflex scapular vessels, which were found to perfuse the muscle instead of the thoracodorsal vessels [333].

Advantages and Disadvantages

The advantages of the latissimus dorsi flap overcome its few disadvantages very clearly: because of its constant vascular anatomy, the high density of myocutaneous perforators to the overlying skin, the relatively long and high-caliber vessels, and because of the ease of flap raising, the latissimus dorsi is a popular and safe flap, offering numerous possibilities for defect cover. Normally, the morbidity of the donor site is low, but can increase with simultaneous radical neck dissection with sacrifice of the accessory nerve. In these circumstances, stability of the shoulder can be reduced [399]. Although a reduction of function and strength of the shoulder generally is not experienced by most patients, some sports activities can be negatively affected [196, 212, 310]. Whereas Laitung and Peck found good compensation of the latissimus function by other muscle groups even in patients who are active in sports [216], Russel and co-workers noted weakness in all muscles surrounding the operated shoulder [321]. The most significant disadvantage of the latissimus dorsi flap is the difficulty of flap raising simultaneous to tumor resection in the head and neck area [15, 286]. When bringing the patient in a lateral decubitus position prior to flap harvesting, care must be taken to stabilize the contralateral shoulder to prevent injury to the brachial plexus [250, 451]; otherwise, weakness or paralysis of the radial nerve [299] or permanent loss of sensitivity [22] or complete loss of motor function [224] in the upper extremity can occur. If the donor site has to be covered by skin grafting, the aesthetic result is always poor, so that flaps should not be outlined wider than 10 cm. [233, 286]. Despite the flat shape of the muscle, the myocutaneous latissimus dorsi flap is often too bulky for small and medium-sized defects of the oral cavity, because a considerable layer of adipose tissue between muscle and skin is found in many patients. When used for facial contour augmentation, the subsequent atrophy of the muscle component can lead to unfavorable secondary volume loss [310].

Flap Raising

Patient Positioning

The patient is brought in a lateral decubitus position and a pad is placed between the shoulder and the neck on the contralateral side to prevent impingement of the brachial plexus by the clavicle. The ipsilateral arm is included in the operating field to allow for free movement, and it is prepped and draped together with the lateral thorax, shoulder, axilla, and back. If the patient is in the prone position, which is also possible for flap raising, reprepping and redraping must be performed before the operation is continued with the patient in the supine position.

Flap Design

Although skin paddles can be designed with a high variability over the entire proximal two-thirds of the muscle, in a standard situation it is highly recommended to outline the skin paddle over its anterior part with the flap axis running 4–5 cm dorsal to the anterior edge of the latissimus dorsi. The anterior border of the skin paddle should not exceed the rim of the muscle, and the flap width should be limited to 10 cm to allow primary closure. For exposure of the pedicle, a straight incision is marked from the proximal pole of the flap to the axilla. Correct placement of the skin paddle must be checked carefully by palpating the anterior muscle rim, which forms the posterior demarcation of the axilla groove. Because of the consistent anatomy of the pedicle and the high number of perforators, no preoperative measures are necessary before flap raising, if no previous surgery (lymphadenectomy) has been performed in the axilla.

The initial incision is made along the anterior border of the skin paddle and continued into the axilla from the upper pole of the flap. The subcutaneous fatty tissue, the amount of which can vary considerably, is transected perpendicularly until the muscle fibers are reached. The anterior rim of the latissimus muscle is exposed by dissecting the fatty tissue away from the serratus muscle and retracting it in an anterior direction. The fat underlying the skin paddle should not be separated from the latissimus muscle.

Step 1

With the anterior border of the latissimus clearly identified, by further retracting the skin and subcutaneous fatty tissue in an anterior direction, a branch of the thoracodorsal artery, which supplies the serratus anterior muscle, is exposed. This strong vessel is the first branch of the thoracodorsal artery, which now becomes visible. The serratus branch is then traced proximally, leading directly to the vascular pedicle. Additionally, the thoracodorsal artery can be located easily by palpating its pulsation underneath the proximal muscle rim.

Step 2

The anterior rim of the muscle is elevated and retracted, so that the vascular pedicle can be dissected. The serratus branch leading to the thoracodorsal vessels is preserved until the end of flap raising. Now the pedicle is dissected in the cranial direction. A second side branch of the thoracodorsal vessels becomes visible opposite the serratus branch, which runs to the inferior angle of the scapula. Depending on the desired pedicle length, the thoracodorsal vessels are followed up to the axilla, until the circumflex scapula vessels are reached. Dissecting caudally, the neurovascular hilum is found about 2–4 cm distal to the serratus branch, where the thoracodorsal vessels enter the muscle at its undersurface. Here, the vein is located lateral to the artery, and the motor nerve runs between the vessels.

Step 3

A vessel loop is placed around the neurovascular pedicle inferior to the serratus and scapula branch, and the latissimus dorsi muscle is further undermined by blunt dissection. Careful hemostasis is necessary, especially in the distal and medial parts, where segmental branches of the lumbar artery also supply the latissimus dorsi muscle.

Step 4

The skin paddle is now completely peritomized to the muscle fascia. The muscle is elevated, and then the muscle fibers are transected along the inferior pole of the flap. Because the anterior border of the skin paddle corresponds to the anterior muscle rim, the muscle must not be transected along the anterior periphery of the flap.

Step 5

The posterior parts of the latissimus muscle can now be elevated easily, and the fibrofatty tissue between the latissimus and the serratus muscle is divided.

Step 6

Step 7   Depending on the dimensions of the skin paddle, the muscle is incised along its posterior periphery. The neurovascular pedicle is slightly retracted from the muscle to precisely visualize the neurovascular hilum in the region of the cranial pole of the flap.

Step 8   The latissimus dorsi now is completely divided cranial to the neurovascular hilum, creating a strip of muscle between the cranial pole of the skin paddle and the vascular hilum, which carries the vertical branch of the thoracodorsal vessels. The horizontal branch running along the superior border of the latissimus dorsi muscle is transected at the cranial flap pole shortly after the bifurcation of the thoracodorsal vessels. To ensure safe protection of the vertical branch, which runs 1.5–3 cm away from the anterior border, this strip of muscle should be about 4–5 cm wide.

Step 9   Finally, the side branches of the thoracodorsal vessels to the serratus muscle and the inferior angle of scapula are divided. The flap is now ready for microvascular transfer. Because of their high caliber, the artery, vein, and nerve can easily be separated from each other. The thoracodorsal nerve can be used for flap reinnervation. Perfusion of the flap is maintained until the recipient vessels are prepared for anastomoses. A drain is inserted, and direct wound closure is achieved after mobilization and hemostasis.

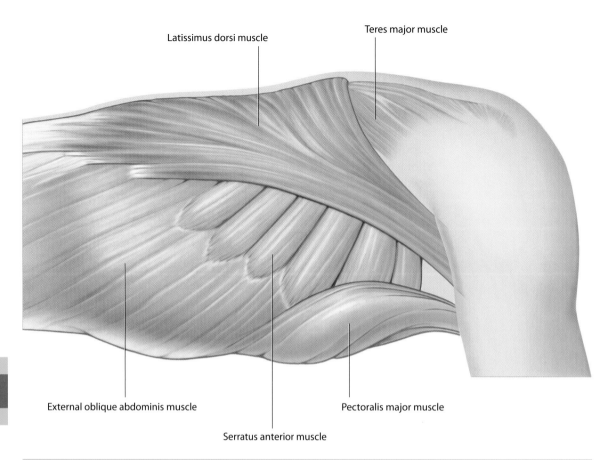

Latissimus dorsi muscle

Teres major muscle

External oblique abdominis muscle

Pectoralis major muscle

Serratus anterior muscle

Muscle anatomy of the lateral thoracic wall

Vascular system and standard flap design along anterior muscle rim ▶

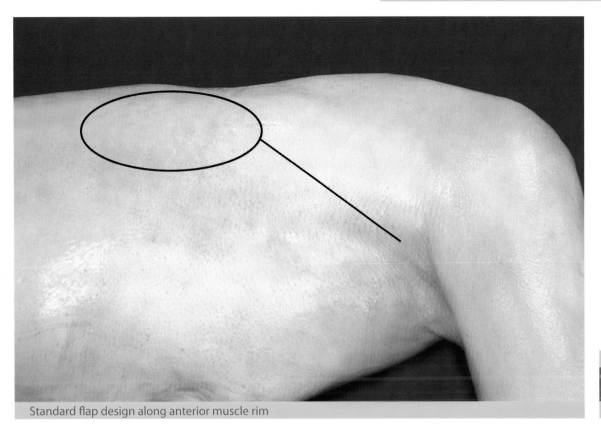

Standard flap design along anterior muscle rim

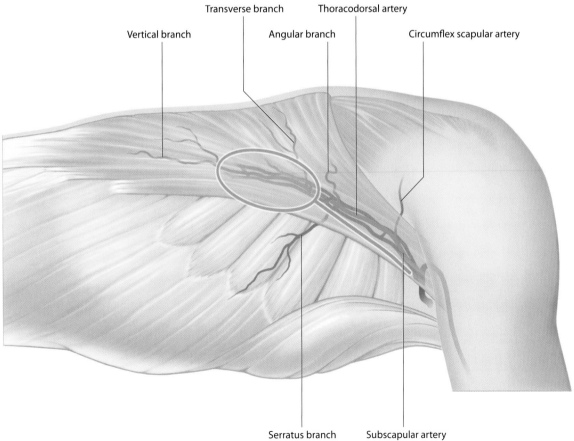

Vertical branch

Transverse branch

Angular branch

Thoracodorsal artery

Circumflex scapular artery

Serratus branch

Subscapular artery

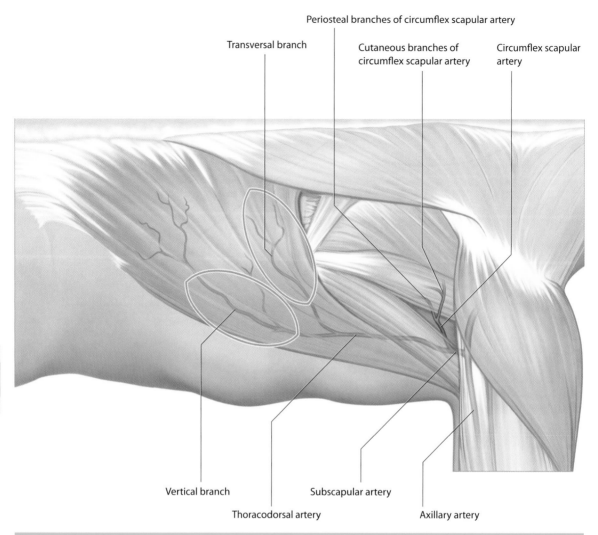

Periosteal branches of circumflex scapular artery

Transversal branch

Cutaneous branches of
circumflex scapular artery

Circumflex scapular
artery

Vertical branch

Thoracodorsal artery

Subscapular artery

Axillary artery

Second skin paddle placed along the transversal branch

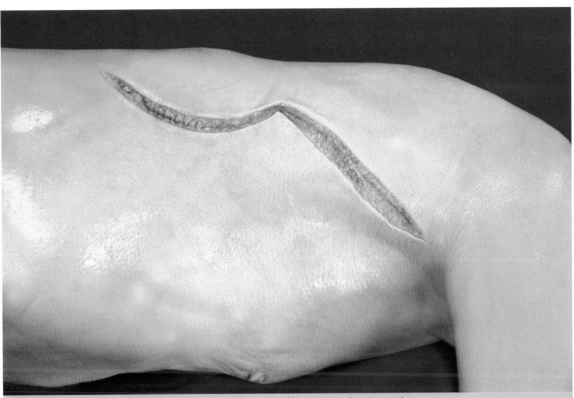

Step 1 • Skin incision and exposure of anterior rim of latissimus dorsi muscle

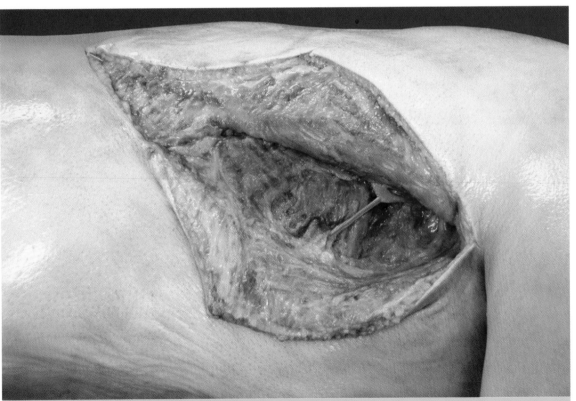

Step 2 • Identification of anterior muscle rim and serratus branch

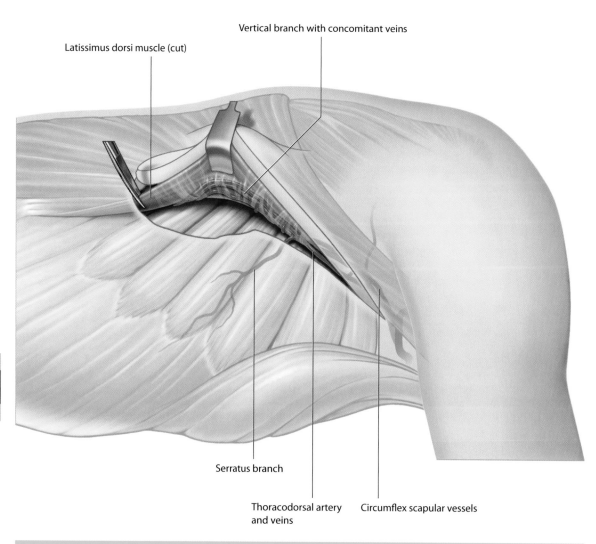

Latissimus dorsi muscle (cut)

Vertical branch with concomitant veins

Serratus branch

Thoracodorsal artery
and veins

Circumflex scapular vessels

Anatomic relation of serratus branch, anterior muscle rim and thoracodorsal vessels

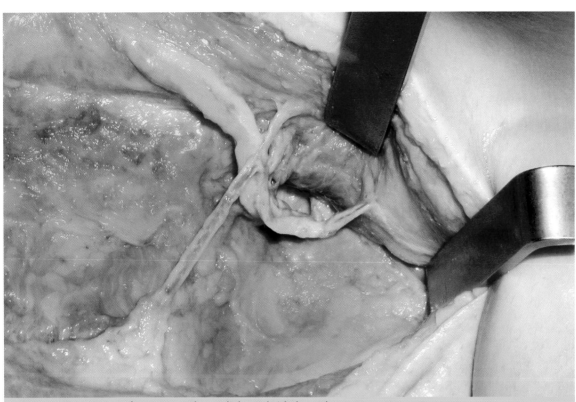

Step 3 • Dissection of neurovascular pedicle and side branches

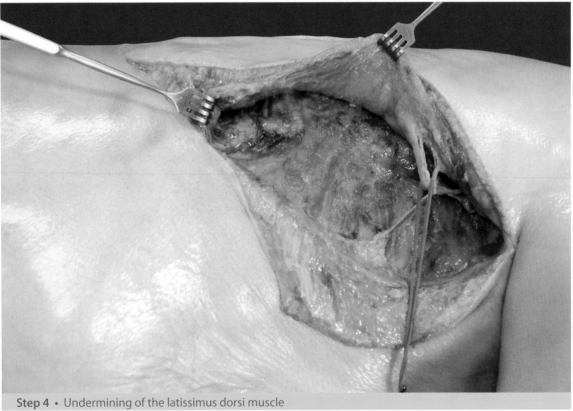

Step 4 • Undermining of the latissimus dorsi muscle

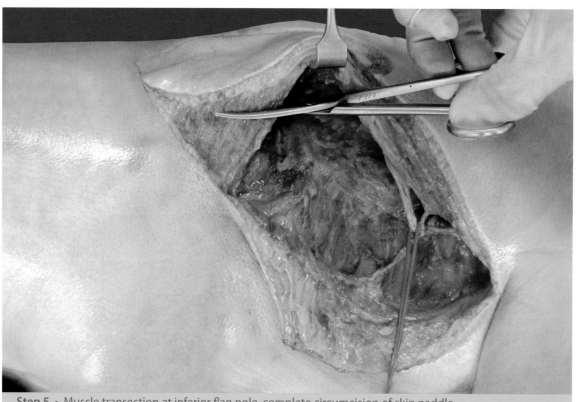

Step 5 • Muscle transection at inferior flap pole, complete circumcision of skin paddle

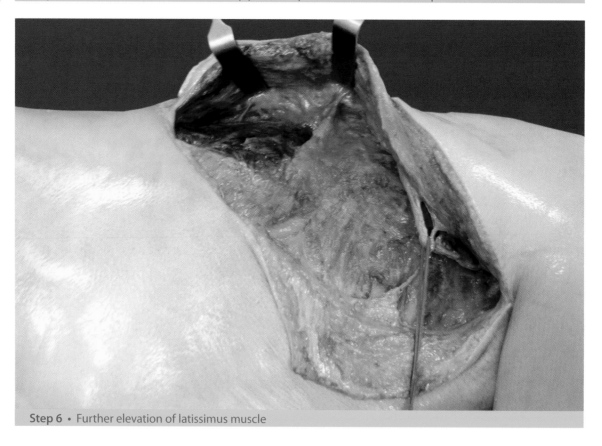

Step 6 • Further elevation of latissimus muscle

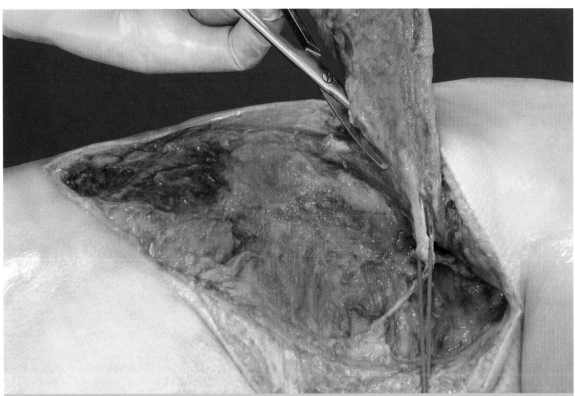

Step 7 • Transecting the latissimus dorsi muscle along the posterior periphery of the flap

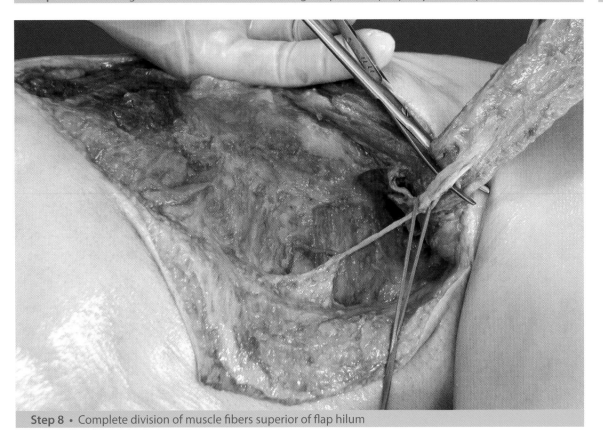

Step 8 • Complete division of muscle fibers superior of flap hilum

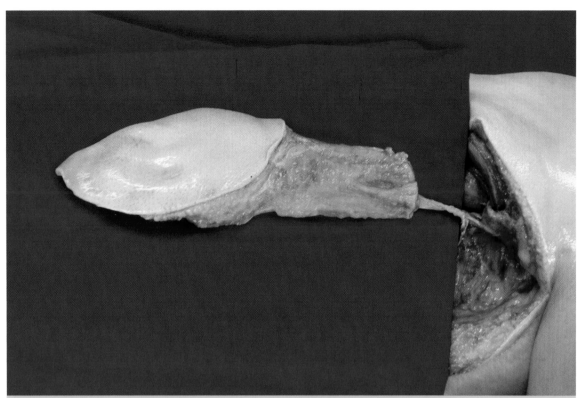

Step 9 • Elevated flap still attached to the neurovascular pedicle

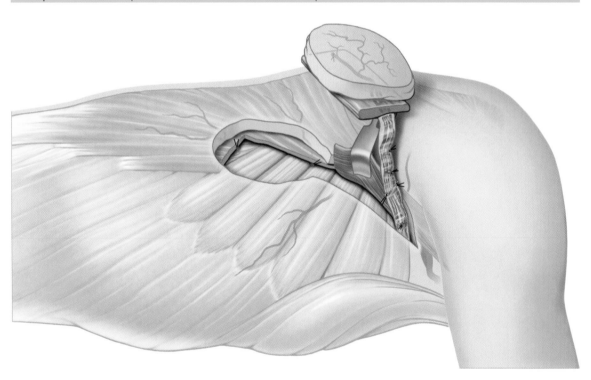

Raised flap containing a dense network of myocutaneous perforators

Comments

Step 1: The anterior border of the latissimus muscle can easily be missed, especially in obese patients. To determine its location, a line is drawn between the dorsal axillary fold and the midline of the iliac crest. In slim patients, the muscle rim can easily be palpated and marked pre-operatively during active adduction of the arm by the patient. Somefew advise first exposing the anterior muscle rim proximal to the skin paddle to exactly determine the position of the anterior flap border, which should not exceed the muscle. To estimate the amount of skin that can be removed and still allow for direct closure, a large fold of skin should be pinched at the flap site.

Step 2: The serratus branch should not be mistaken for the thoracodorsal artery. Do not transect or ligate this vessel before the thoracodorsal artery is clearly identified.

Step 3: Proximal dissection of the vascular pedicle is facilitated if the skin incision is extended to the onset of the posterior axillary fold. At the level of the circumflex scapular vessels, the length of the thoracodorsal artery to the neurovascular hilum of the flap is at least 7 cm.

Step 5: To prevent shearing forces to the perforating vessels, the skin paddle should be fixed to the muscle with stay sutures.

Step 7: If the strip of muscle is too narrow, the vertical branch of the thoracodorsal artery may be missed. One should be aware that flap raising is facilitated and more reliable if the muscle component has nearly the same size as the skin paddle.

Step 8: Clearly visualize the neurovascular hilum before the muscle is peritomized cranially.

Step 9: Do not remove the stay sutures between the skin paddle and the muscle until the flap is fixed at the recipient site. If the vascular pedicle is not dissected up to subscapular artery, the larger of the two veins should be used for anastomosis.

Scapular Flap

Chapter 5

Wolff/Hölzle, *Raising of Microvascular Flaps 2nd ed.*,
DOI: 10.1007/978-3-642-13831-7_5, © Springer-Verlag Berlin Heidelberg 2011

Development and Indications

The subscapular vascular system and its suitability for flap harvesting first was investigated in an anatomic study by Saijo in 1978 [326]. Two years later, Dos Santos made use of these anatomical findings [92]. He described the scapular flap as a lipocutaneous flap, nourished by a transverse septocutaneous branch from the circumflex scapular artery. This flap, the axis of which was oriented inferior and parallel to the scapular spine, was successfully transferred by Gilbert in 1979 [120]. Following further, more detailed anatomical studies [121, 251, 386], a number of clinical series were reported using this flap, which soon was accepted as another useful tool for coverage of soft tissue defects [23, 123, 138, 391, 397]. A variation of this flap was described in 1982 by Nassif and co-workers, who proposed using the descending septocutaneous branch of the circumflex scapular artery as the vessel nourishing the skin [280]. Thus they designed the skin paddle of this parascapular flap along the lateral border of the scapula. Already in 1981, Teot and co-workers published that from an anatomical point of view all preconditions are fulfilled to build a purely osseous flap from the scapula bone [386]. Nevertheless, it was not until 1986 when harvesting osteocutaneous flaps by including the lateral border of the scapula was popularized [356, 372]. Since that time, the indications for flaps raised from the scapular donor site have been considerably expanded [19, 99, 356, 372]. Since the vascular pedicle develops from the same source artery like the latissimus dorsi flap, both flaps can be combined using only one set of anastomoses at the subscapular vessels [279]. The spectrum of indications for flaps raised from the scapular region, in the head and neck area, ranges from contour augmentations using deepithelialized adipofascial flaps to closure of extended perforating composite defects with simultaneous mandible reconstruction using osteomyocutaneous scapular and latissimus dorsi flaps [19, 76, 77, 178, 305, 310, 396]. Moreover, a number of useful applications were soon described for defect cover in the upper [50, 109, 158] and lower extremities [58, 80, 121, 199, 348, 397].

Anatomy

The circumflex scapular artery is one of the two main branches of the subscapularis artery, which has a diameter of 3–4 mm at its origin from the distal third of the axillaris artery [233]. During its course to the scapula region, the artery, which is accompanied by two comitant veins, has to penetrate the posterior triangle. This triangle is built by the teres muscles and the long head of the triceps. After giving off small branches to the surrounding muscles, the circumflex scapula artery divides into a deep and a superficial branch, the first of which runs underneath the teres major muscle and divides into terminal branches to reach the periosteum of the lateral border of the scapula bone. The blood supply to the periosteum of the scapula was investigated by Coleman and Sultan [76]. According to their findings, an angular branch, nourishing the tip of the scapula, arose from the thoracodorsal artery just proximal to the serratus branch in 58% of cases, so that the tip of the scapula can be transferred to the thoracodorsal vessels as well. This angular branch first was described by Deraemacher et al., who reported on the possibility of transferring the tip of the scapula together with the serratus anterior muscle on the thoracodorsal artery [90]. In a detailed anatomical study, the angular branch was found to run between the serratus, subscapular, and teres major muscle to the inferior angle of the scapula. The second main branch, the superficial branch of the circumflex scapular artery, divides into the transverse and descending cutaneous branch to perfuse the scapular and the parascapular skin flap, respectively. Whereas in more than 100 cadaver dissections the transverse branch has been found to always be present, with a diameter of 1.5–2.5 mm [93, 121, 397], Godina was unable to identify this cutaneous vessel in three of 28 clinical cases [123]. When raising the skin paddle as a scapular flap, the flap axis is outlined below and parallel to the spine of scapula. According to Urbaniak et al., the limits of the skin paddle should be 2 cm below the scapular spine, 2 cm above the angle, and 2 cm lateral to the midline [397]. Although in an anatomical dissection it was shown that the vascular tree passes the midline and reaches the contralateral acromion [166], Hamilton pointed out that the maximum length of a scapula skin paddle should not be more than 24 cm and should not reach the midline because of the risk of necrosis of the tip of the skin island [138]. By additionally anastomosing the flap to the contralateral circumflex scapular artery, a 50×10-cm biscapular flap can be harvested [24, 102]. When planning a parascapular skin island, the flap axis is oriented above the lateral scapular border, which can be 25 cm long [68] or even 30 cm [350]. Because the terminal branches to the skin form a dense network of anastomoses, building a subdermal and epifascial vascular plexus, fasciosubcutaneous and deep subcutaneous flap compartments can separately be transferred and used for contour augmentations [112, 396]. The length of the vascular pedicle depends on the extent of proximal dissection. If the vascular pedicle is limited to the circumflex scapular artery, its maximum length will be 7–10 cm. Lengthening the pedicle up to 11–14 cm is possible by including the subscapular vessels, transecting these vessels at their point of takeoff from the axillary artery and vein [280]. The circumflex scapular artery is joined by two comitant veins, between 2.5 and 4 mm in diameter. In the majority of cases, these veins unify with the thoracodorsal vein or, which is the case in 10%, enter the axillary vein separately [93].

Advantages and Disadvantages

The major advantages of the scapular skin flap become obvious when comparing it with the osteocutaneous flaps of other donor sites: the skin of the scapular flap is for the most part hairless and similar to the facial skin in texture and color. It carries only a thin layer of adipose tissue, and primary closure of the donor site is possible up to a flap width of 8–10 cm. Moreover, the vascular pedicle can be dissected to an acceptable length and has a high caliber. There are only very few anatomical variations concerning the vascular pedicle, and flap design can be variable. The possibility to simultaneously raise latissimus dorsi [279] or parascapular flaps, which all can be left pedicled at the same source artery, further broadens the spectrum of indications [356, 372]. Up to four flap components can be created, each of them offering the possibility for free and independent positioning [294, 310]. Because of the specific architecture of the scapula, the maxilla can be reconstructed using the blade of the bone to replace the hard palate [178, 310, 399]. Primary closure of the donor site defect is for the most part possible even following harvesting of wide flaps, but unacceptable broad scars can result if tensionless wound closure is impossible [233]. Raising combined scapular and parascapular flaps is always limited by the ability to achieve direct closure [310]. To avoid the application of skin grafts, pretransfer expansion of the skin has been performed in suitable cases [396]. By prelaminating the bone with dermis and simultaneous insertion of enosseous implants, reconstructions of the alveolar ridge with a mucosa-like surface are possible [339], and raising an additional skin flap can be avoided. Even after harvest of osteocutaneous flaps, which makes transection of the teres muscles necessary, disability of the shoulder is reported to be low [77, 294, 399]. Postoperative care includes immobilization of the arm for 3–4 days and physiotherapy to strengthen the muscles of the shoulder girdle, starting about 2–3 weeks after surgery. The main disadvantage of the scapular donor site is given by the fact that simultaneous flap raising is impossible when tumor resections in the head and neck area have to be carried out. In these cases, flap harvesting cannot be started until tumor resection is completed, resulting in a considerable time loss; additionally, new positioning and reprepping of the patient is time-consuming. Whereas identification of the cutaneous branches is normally achieved quickly, dissection of the vascular pedicle by working through the posterior triangle can become difficult in the raising of cutaneous flaps, especially if a long pedicle is needed [98]. To simplify dissection of the vascular pedicle, Gahhos et al. proposed performing a second incision at the axilla, which facilitates identification of the subscapular vessels [113]. Then the flap can be pulled towards the axilla to obtain maximum pedicle length.

Flap Raising

Patient Positioning

Flap elevation is performed with the patient in the prone or lateral decubitus position. The shoulder, back, lateral thorax, and upper arm are circularly prepped to allow for movement of the extremity and exposure of the subscapular system from an axillary approach, if needed. In the lateral decubitus position, bags are used to stabilize the patient and to protect the dependent shoulder. Preoperatively, the location of the circumflex scapular artery (CSA) is identified using a Doppler in the triangular space at the lateral rim of the scapula. Due to constant anatomy, angiography is only necessary if operative procedures at the donor site (axillary lymphadenectomy) have been performed previously.

Flap Design

Skin paddles can be elevated along the axis of the transverse (scapular flap) or descending branch (parascapular flap) of the CSA. In the standard situation, a scapular flap is outlined, keeping the upper, lower, and medial margins of the flap at least 2 cm away from the scapular spine, inferior angle and posterior midline. The angle, spine, and lateral border of the scapula have to be palpated before outlining the flap. For both the scapular and the parascapular flap, it is critical to outline the lateral part of the skin paddle safely above the triangular space, where the CSA runs along the fascial septum between the teres major and minor muscles to enter the posterior thoracic fascia and the skin. This triangular space is found either by palpation of the muscular groove lateral to the scapular bone or, more exactly, by preoperative mapping of the artery using a Doppler. The width of the flap may not exceed 8–10 cm to allow for direct closure. The bone segment is harvested from the lateral scapular border, inferior to the glenohumeral joint and mostly including the inferior angle.

Step 1 Starting medially, skin and subcutaneous fatty tissue are incised to the deep fascia overlying the infraspinatus muscle. The fascia, which consists of multiple layers, is included at the undersurface of the flap, but the deepest layer of fascia, directly covering the muscle fibers, is left intact.

Step 2 The dissection proceeds to the lateral direction by bluntly separating the fasciocutaneous flap from the infraspinatus and teres minor muscles, until the posterior muscle triangle is reached. Here, the position of the CSA has already been marked at the skin preoperatively using a Doppler. The pulsation of the cutaneous branch, which is enveloped into the fascia, can now be seen and palpated easily. After the cutaneous branch has been exposed, the skin paddle is peritomized at its lateral portion and completely elevated.

Now the CSA is traced proximally and the fascial space between the teres minor and major muscles is opened. The lateral margin of scapula is identified by retracting the teres minor medially to expose the perforators to the bone, branching off from the deep segment of the CSA. A vessel loop is placed around the CSA proximal to the bone feeders, which are carefully protected during further flap raising.

Step 3

In the close-up view, the deep segment of the CSA is visible, giving off three branches to the proximal lateral border of the scapula. The cutaneous branch courses directly into the undersurface of the skin paddle, where it divides into the horizontal (scapula skin paddle) and the descending branch (parascapular skin paddle).

Step 4

To gain access to the scapular bone, the infraspinatus muscle is incised 3 cm parallel to the lateral border of scapula, leaving a muscle cuff attached to the bone. The muscle is transected completely, starting at the inferior angle of scapula and ending cranial to the bone feeders.

Step 5

Cranial to the branches of the CSA to the bone, the teres minor and infraspinatus muscles are transected perpendicular to the muscle fibers to prepare for the osteotomy.

Step 6

86

The teres major, which originates from the inferior angle and lateral rim of scapula, is separated from the latissimus dorsi at the inferior angle, and the caudal portion of scapula is undermined.

Step 7

The teres major is now elevated and undermined, so that the angular branch of the thoracodorsal artery becomes visible. Although this vessel contributes to the blood supply of the tip region, it can be transected without endangering the viability of the scapular bone flap. If an isolated angular bone segment is planned, the vascular pedicle should include the thoracodorsal artery, and the angular branch is left intact.

Step 8

The teres major muscle is now transected directly at the lateral border of the scapula. Doing this, the vascular branches of the CSA to the bone must be protected carefully.

Step 9

The osteotomy is performed, beginning 1–2 cm inferior of the glenohumeral joint. Here, care must be taken not to injure the vascular pedicle. The osteotomy is normally carried out 2–3 cm parallel to the lateral border of the scapula and can include the entire inferior angle.

Step 10

After completion of the osteotomy, the bone segment remains attached to the subscapularis and teres minor muscles. Retracting the scapular bone segment laterally, the subscapular muscle becomes visible at the undersurface of the scapula and is divided in a distal to cranial direction.

Step 11

Step 12   Residual muscular attachments are identified at the vascular hilum of the bone segment, and the remaining fibers of the subscapularis muscle are divided.

Step 13   The bone flap can now be elevated further, so that transection of the remaining fibers of the teres minor muscle is possible without endangering the CSA and its branches.

Step 14   The osteocutaneous scapular flap is now completely elevated and ready for microvascular transfer. To lengthen the vascular pedicle, the CSA can be traced to the subscapular artery. Exposure of the subscapular artery is facilitated via an additional approach through the axilla, but this is rarely necessary. To prevent scapula winging, the teres major muscle is reattached by drill holes in the lateral border of the residual scapula. A deep drain is inserted, and wound closure is accomplished after wide undermining. Postoperatively, the shoulder is immobilized for 1 week.

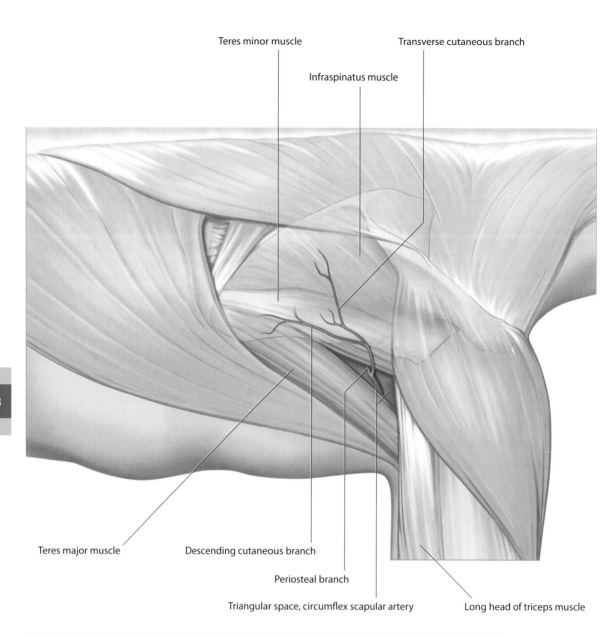

Teres minor muscle

Infraspinatus muscle

Transverse cutaneous branch

Teres major muscle

Descending cutaneous branch

Periosteal branch

Triangular space, circumflex scapular artery

Long head of triceps muscle

Muscle and vascular anatomy of the scapular donor site

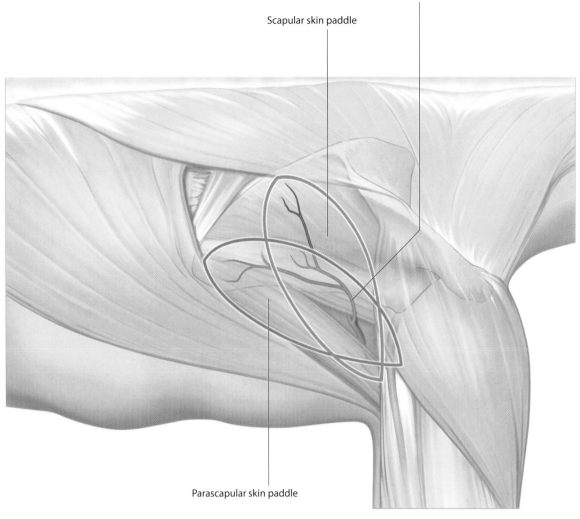

Circumflex scapular artery, cutaneous branches

Scapular skin paddle

Parascapular skin paddle

Design of scapular and parascapular skin paddle

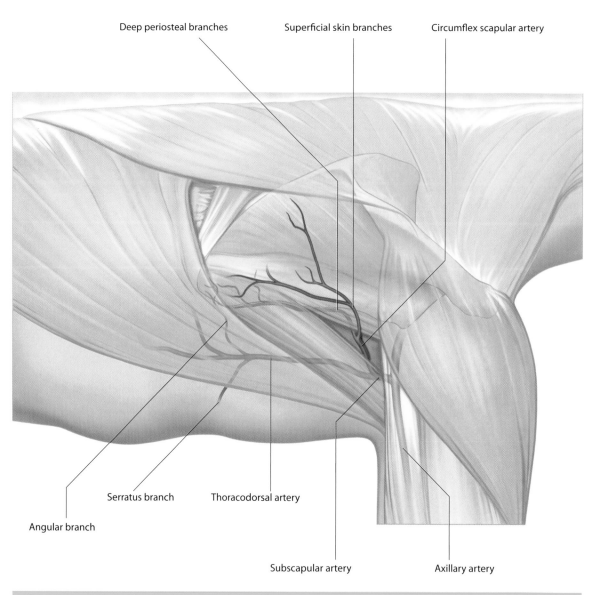

Deep periosteal branches

Superficial skin branches

Circumflex scapular artery

Serratus branch

Thoracodorsal artery

Angular branch

Subscapular artery

Axillary artery

Vascular system developing from the subscapularis artery

90

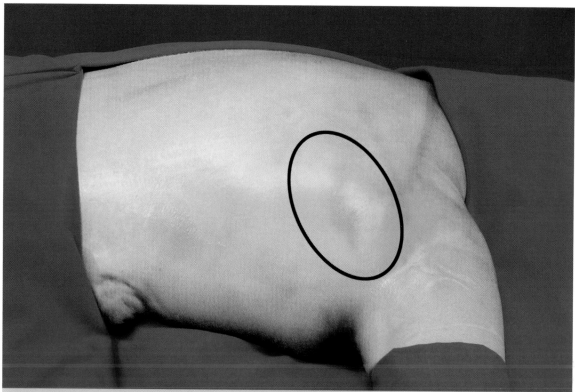

Standard design of scapular skin paddle

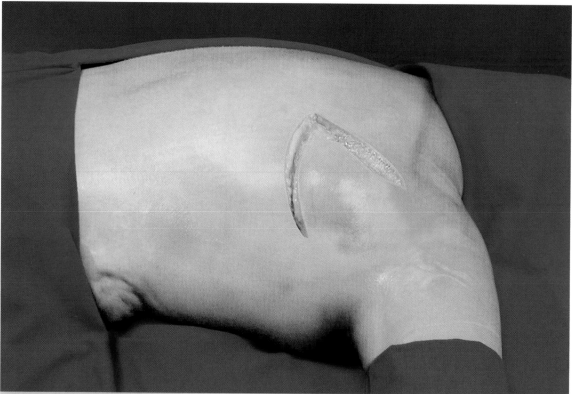

Step 1 • Circumcision of medial pole of scapular skin paddle to the deep fascia

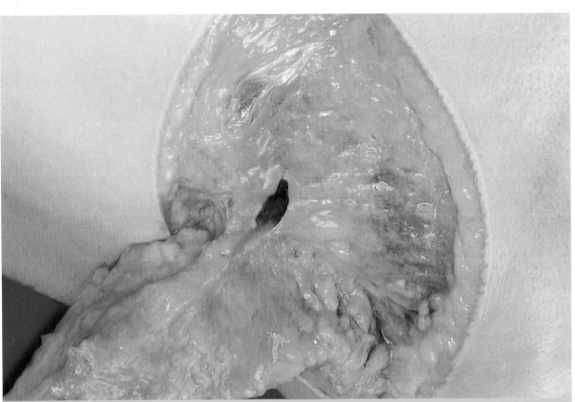

Step 2 • Identification of superficial branch of the circumflex scapular artery (CSA)

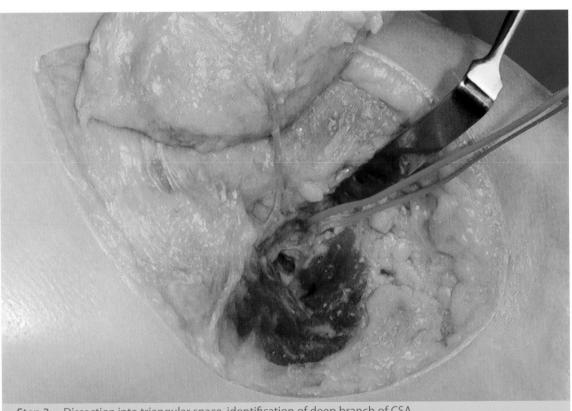

Step 3 • Dissection into triangular space, identification of deep branch of CSA

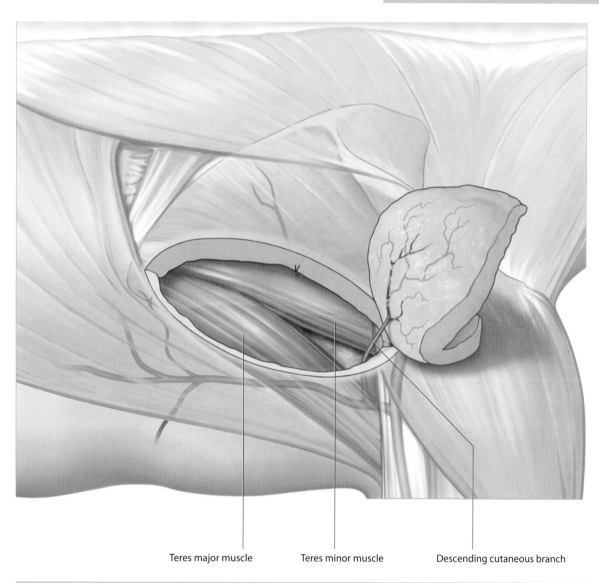

Teres major muscle   Teres minor muscle   Descending cutaneous branch

Elevation of parascapular skin paddle

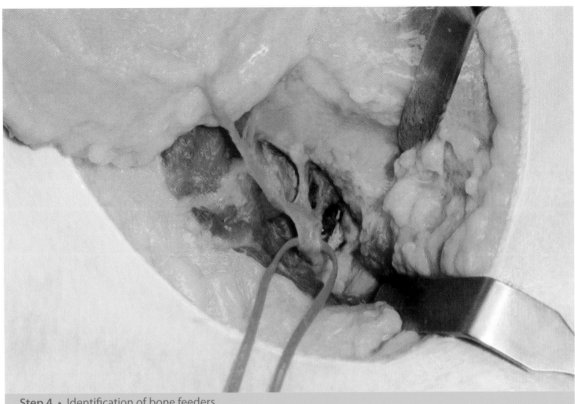

Step 4 • Identification of bone feeders

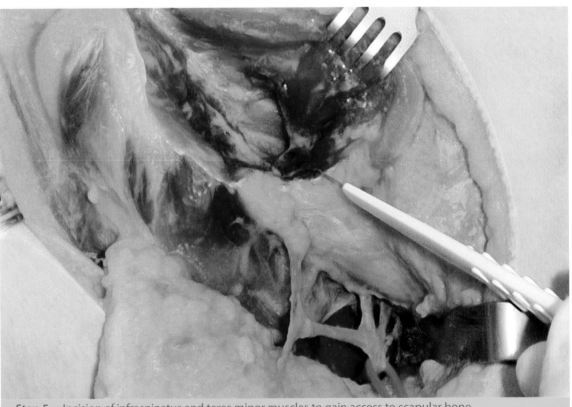

Step 5 • Incision of infraspinatus and teres minor muscles to gain access to scapular bone

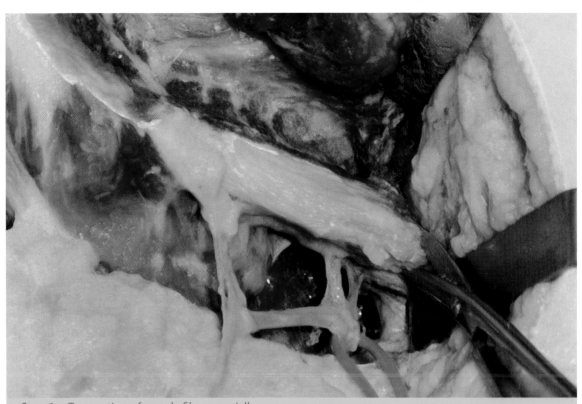

Step 6 • Transection of muscle fibers cranially

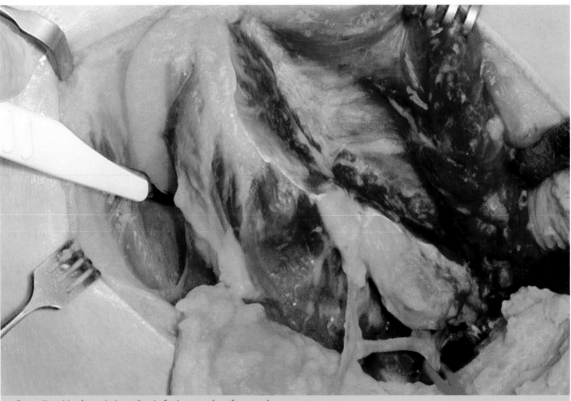

Step 7 • Undermining the inferior angle of scapula

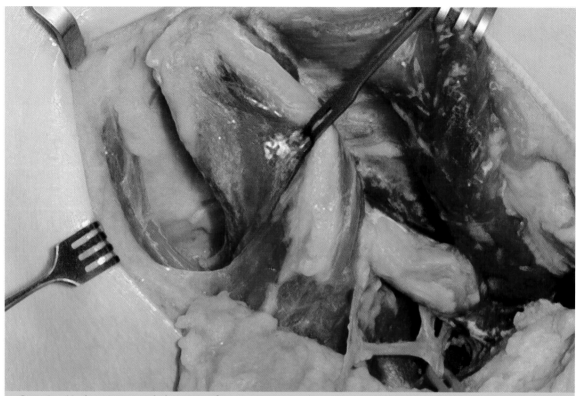

Step 8 • Undermining and elevation of teres major muscle

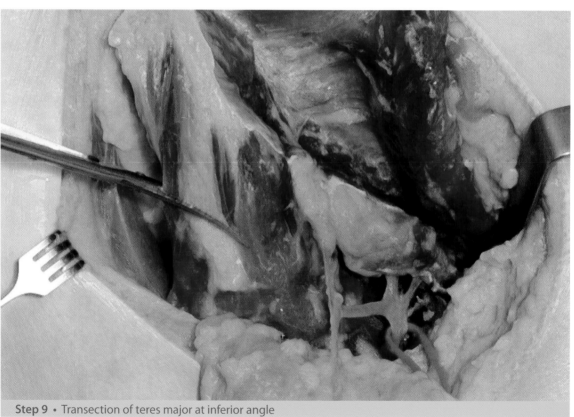

Step 9 • Transection of teres major at inferior angle

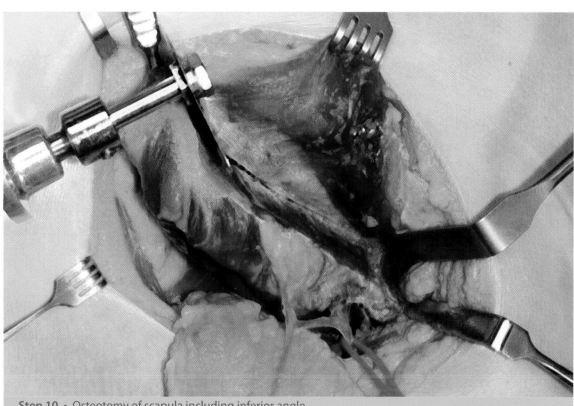

Step 10 • Osteotomy of scapula including inferior angle

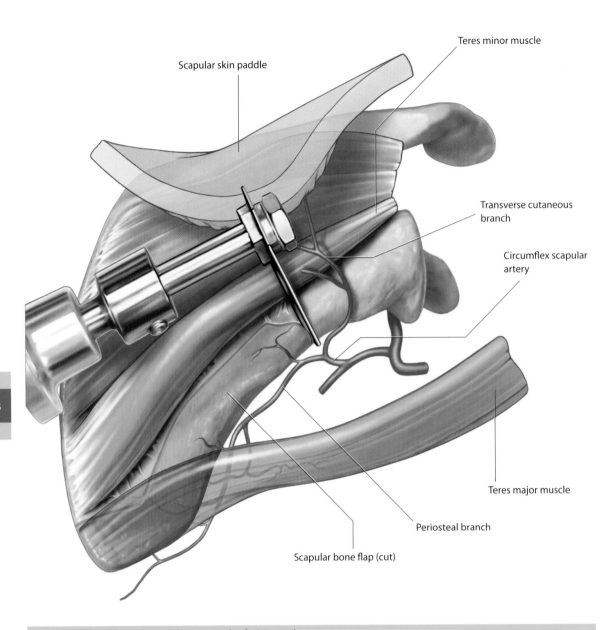

Scapular skin paddle

Teres minor muscle

Transverse cutaneous branch

Circumflex scapular artery

Teres major muscle

Periosteal branch

Scapular bone flap (cut)

Osteotomy of lateral scapular rim and inferior angle

98

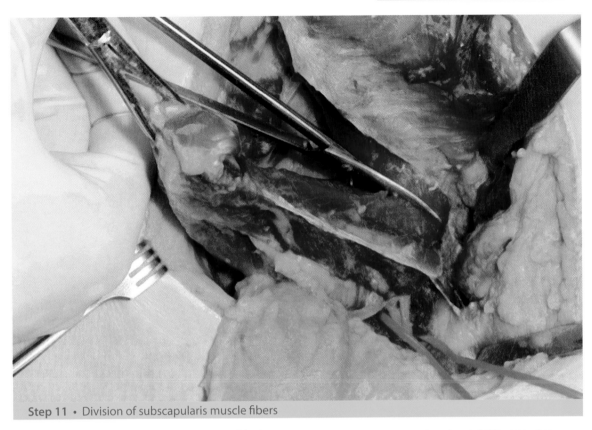

Step 11 • Division of subscapularis muscle fibers

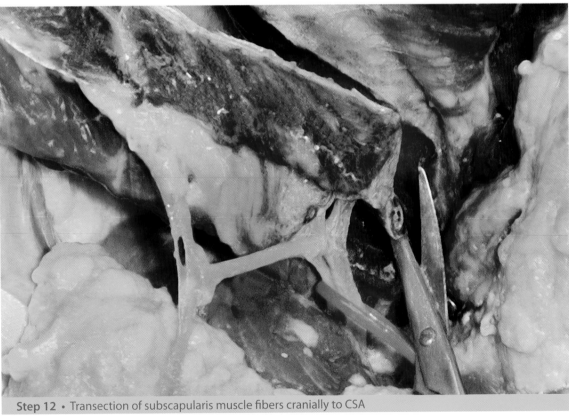

Step 12 • Transection of subscapularis muscle fibers cranially to CSA

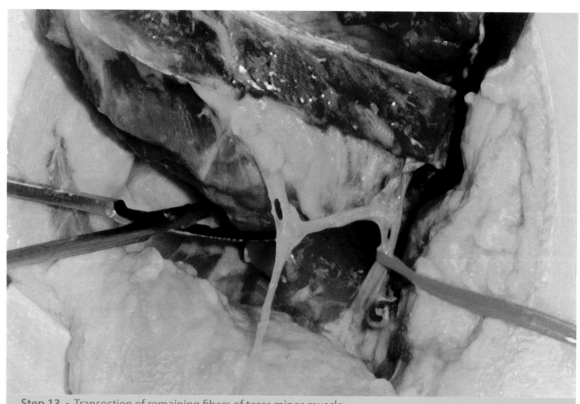

Step 13 • Transection of remaining fibers of teres minor muscle

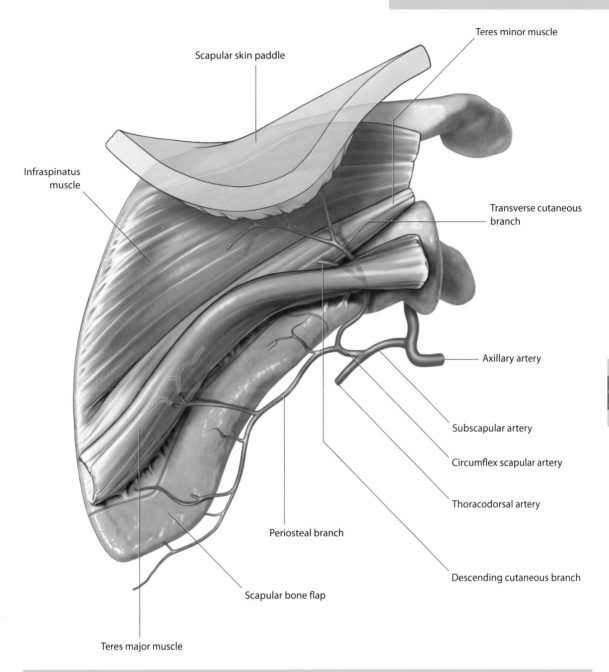

Scapular skin paddle

Teres minor muscle

Infraspinatus muscle

Transverse cutaneous branch

Axillary artery

Subscapular artery

Circumflex scapular artery

Thoracodorsal artery

Periosteal branch

Descending cutaneous branch

Scapular bone flap

Teres major muscle

Vascular anatomy of the osteocutaneous scapular flap

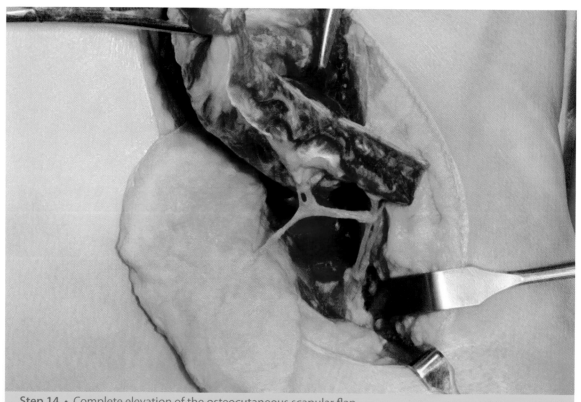

Step 14 • Complete elevation of the osteocutaneous scapular flap

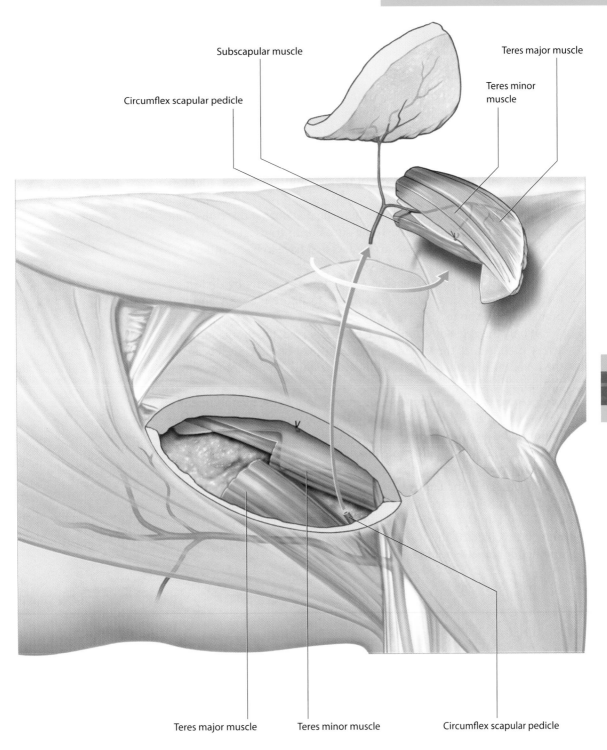

Subscapular muscle

Circumflex scapular pedicle

Teres major muscle

Teres minor muscle

Teres major muscle

Teres minor muscle

Circumflex scapular pedicle

Raised osteocutaneous scapular flap and donor-site defect

Comments

Planning

In obese patients, palpation of the triangular space between the teres minor and major and the long head of triceps can be difficult. In these patients, Doppler sonography is mandatory to determine the lateral pole of the skin paddle.

Step 1: Do not define the lateral pole of the flap until the CSA is identified.

Step 3: Many muscular branches have to be ligated during dissection of the deep segment of the CSA. To be sure not to transect one of the branches to the bone, the osseous feeders first have to be identified at the lateral margin of the scapula.

Steps 4–9: When preparing the scapula for the osteotomy by dividing the muscle fibers, care must be taken not to injure the CSA and its branches to the bone.

Step 8: If only the angle of scapula is to be transferred, the thoracodorsal artery is chosen as the vascular pedicle instead of the CSA, because the tip of the scapula is nourished by the scapular branch of the thoracodorsal artery.

Step 10: Do not extend the bone segment too close to the glenohumeral joint, where the thickness of the scapular bone is markedly increased. Injury to the joint will lead to significant dysfunction of the shoulder.

Steps 10–13: The skin paddle, which has already been elevated, must be protected from shearing strains while handling the bone segment. The superficial branch and all branches to the scapular bone must be observed during transection of the residual adherent muscle fibers.

Step 1, 2, 14: Direct closure of the donor site under excessive tension must be avoided. If the width of the skin paddle exceeds 8–10 cm, another donor site should be considered.

Fibular Flap

Wolff/Hölzle, *Raising of Microvascular Flaps 2nd ed.*,
DOI: 10.1007/978-3-642-13831-7_6, © Springer-Verlag Berlin Heidelberg 2011

Development and Indications

The first microvascular bone transfer was performed by Taylor and co-workers, who used a vascularized myo-osseous segment of the fibula for treatment of a post-traumatic defect of the tibia in 1975 [382]. Since this first description, the primary indications for the fibular bone flap have been reconstructions of extended bone defects in the extremities using a posterior approach for flap harvesting, which was originally described by Taylor et al. [382]. Whereas these first transfers of the fibula were performed without including a skin paddle, Chen and Yan were the first to report an osteocutaneous fibula flap in 1983 [64]. This extension of flap raising became possible following the proposal of Gilbert to use a lateral approach for harvesting the bone flap, which was easier to perform and allowed for visualization of the cutaneous branches of the peroneal artery [120]. A valuable extension of the indicational spectrum of the fibular flap was achieved by the report of Hidalgo, who performed the first lower jaw reconstruction using osteotomies to mimic the shape of a nearly entire mandible in 1989 [152]. Since that time, the fibula flap has proven to be a valuable method for mandible reconstruction, especially in extended defects, exceeding the length of half a mandible [64, 110, 152, 227, 334, 349, 416, 431]. By inclusion of the soleus muscle, which was then connected to motor branches at the recipient site, restoration of motor function was achieved [71]. Because of the bone length and the potential to vary the position of the skin paddle, it is possible to combine bone segments and skin islands from different parts of the flap, allowing more flexibility in flap design [418, 425, 431]. Moreover, two separate skin paddles can be harvested and used for closure of through-and-through defects of the cheek, simultaneously reconstructing the mandible using the fibula bone [110, 152, 418, 431]. To overcome the limited height of the fibula, Jones introduced the possibility of folding two osteotomized bone segments over each other [177]. This "double-barreled" fibular flap was first used for reconstruction of segmental defects of the femur, until this method was adapted to mandible reconstruction. To restore sensation of the skin paddle, Hayden and O'Leary harvested the sural cutaneous nerve together with the skin island and anastomosed this nerve to sensitive nerves of the oral cavity [147]. Sensate fibular flaps later were used for penile reconstruction as well [324]. Flap combinations were performed by anastomosing a second free flap to the distal peroneal artery and vein, which do not significantly reduce in caliber and thus can also serve as donor vessels at the recipient site [416].

Anatomy

The dominant vascular pedicle of the fibular flap is the peroneal artery, which develops from the posterior tibial artery. Together with the tibial anterior artery it is one of the three main branches of the popliteal artery. Accompanied by two veins, the lateral of which is usually larger [135], the peroneal artery runs distally between the flexor hallucis longus and tibialis posterior muscles and, in addition to the muscular branches, gives rise to several periosteal and medullary branches to the fibula bone as well as a number of cutaneous perforators, running along the posterior intermuscular septum to the skin of the lateral calf. Normally, the peroneal artery does not significantly contribute to the blood supply of the foot, but due to a number of anatomic variations concerning the tibial anterior or posterior vessels, the peroneal artery can become a dominant nutrient vessel to the foot. According to the anatomic literature, the tibial anterior and posterior vessels can only be rudimentarily present or completely missing [114, 118, 127, 151, 164, 167, 173, 219, 266, 298], so that preoperative angiography or magnetic resonance tomography have to be performed to evaluate the vascular anatomy of the donor site [382, 425, 431, 447]. If one of the three main arteries is significantly reduced in caliber or missing, no flap raising should be performed in this leg. Additionally, atherosclerotic changes will lead to an increased risk for flap loss and possibly long-term ischemic complications at the donor site will occur, so that in these cases another donor site should be considered. Although the venous anatomy was found to be unique in every individual, no contraindications were found from a venous standpoint to raise fibula flaps. The two venae comitantes do not necessarily coalesce into a single common peroneal vein, but in 66% of individuals, they unify to a common peroneal vein and can be lengthened up to the confluence with the popliteal vein. Nevertheless, because of certain anatomical exceptions, the choice of donor vein and venous pedicle length should depend on the anatomy presenting intraoperatively [135]. Although the fibular bone is non-weightbearing, 7- to 8-cm segments must be preserved at the proximal and distal ends during flap raising to protect the common peroneal nerve at the fibular neck and prevent instability of the ankle. Despite this limitation, up to 25 cm of bone length can be harvested, which are enough to restore subtotal or even total mandibular defects [120, 152]. For osteocutaneous transfer of the fibular flap, the location and course of the cutaneous perforators is of particular interest. Clinical experience and anatomical studies conducted to evaluate the reliability of the blood supply to the skin have shown that the cutaneous perforators of the peroneal artery vary in location, course, size, and number. Therefore, different survival rates of the skin paddle have been reported and different proposals have been made to improve the reliability of the fibular flap skin island. Hidalgo, who performed five osteocutaneous fibula transfers in his first series of 12 patients, reported four complete or partial losses and only one complete survival of the skin paddle [152]. To increase the number of cutaneous perforators and thus the safety of skin perfusion, he therefore suggested always including the entire posterior intermuscular septum, independent of the size of the skin paddle [154]. Because of the anatomical variations of the perforating vessels, Urken [398] considered loss rates between 7 and 10% to be inevitable [398]. In an anatomic study on 52 cadavers, Chen et al. found four to seven cutaneous branches, most of them having a myocutaneous course and perforating the soleus muscle [64]. Another description of the cutaneous arteries was given by Yoshimura et al., who differentiated myocutaneous perforators, running through the peroneal muscles, septomyocutaneous perforators, running between the peroneus and soleus muscles and giving off further muscular branches, and purely septocutaneous vessels [447]. A different classification was proposed by Wei and co-workers, who only distinguished septocutaneous perforators, traversing the whole intermuscular posterior septum, and musculocutaneous perforators, additionally coursing through either the peroneus, tibialis posterior, or soleus muscle [416]. In a later publication, these authors reported a 100% survival rate of the skin paddle in more than 100 patients by centering the skin paddle over the transition of the middle and distal third of the fibula [418]. Contrary to Wei's findings, Carriquiry only identified septocutaneous perforators in their ten anatomical dissections [54]; this was supported by Carr and co-workers[51], who stated that the cutaneous perfusion is exclusively maintained by septocutaneous vessels. In an extensive anatomical dissection on 80 cadavers and supported by their clinical experience on 18 patients, Schusterman et al. found a mean 3.7 cutaneous perforating vessels from the peroneal artery, 1.3 of these with a septocutaneous, 1.9 a myocutaneous course, and 0.6 showed a direct adhesion on the muscle fascia without penetrating the muscles [343]. Because of this variability, the authors proposed always including a cuff of tibialis posterior and soleus muscles on either side of the septum for safety reasons. A similar suggestion had already been made in 1986 by Harrison, who improved his success rate with the skin paddle using this method [142]. Nevertheless, Van Twisk considered the inclusion of a muscle cuff to be necessary only if no septocutaneous vessels could be visualized [406]. In his anatomical study on 80 cadavers, Yoshimura, who gave the first description on the peroneal flap [446], which is nourished by the same cutaneous vessels as the osteocutaneous fibula flap, found an average of 4.8 cutaneous vessels, 71% of which had a myocutaneous course to the skin [445]. Whereas he believed that the skin paddle should be designed at the junction of the middle and distal third of the fibula, other authors proposed centering the flap 2 cm superior to the midpoint between the fibula head and ankle [64, 233, 342, 369] and subfascial incision [110]. If no septocutaneous vessels are identified, part of the soleus muscle has to be included to capture the myocutaneous perforators [110]. Based on an anatomical study by Wolff, a mean 4.2 cutaneous perforators were found, most of them with a myocutaneous course through the tibialis posterior and soleus muscles proximally and a septocutaneous course at the distal lower leg [425]. The most reliable region to build a skin paddle turned out to be 8–12 cm proximal to the ankle, because here a strong perforator, mostly having a septocutaneous pattern, was found in all 50 cadavers. As a consequence of these anatomical findings, the author proposed routinely designing the skin paddle at the junction between the medial and the distal third of the fibula, additionally offering the possibility of dissecting a long vascular pedicle. Depending on the length of the bone segment needed and the level on which the peroneal artery unifies with the tibial posterior vessels, the vascular pedicle can reach up to 15 cm, if the skin paddle is raised distally [421, 425, 431]. To obtain a long pedicle, Hidalgo proposed removing the longest fibula segment possible and then discharging the proximal bone segment after having dissected the pedicle together with the surrounding soft tissues in a subperiosteal plane [153]. The blood supply to the distal fibula segment is not altered by this maneuver. Dye injections have been carried out to determine the territory of skin available for the osteocutaneous fibula transfer. When injecting proximally into the peroneal artery, a skin territory approximately 10 cm in width and 20 cm in length is stained, allowing to transfer nearly the entire skin of the lateral calf. Raising such a large skin paddle was considered problematic because of the extensive donor site skin defect. Therefore, other authors proposed raising large skin flaps from an additional donor site or using another osteocutaneous flap [227, 418]. Selective injection studies have shown that a skin territory of about 12×7cm is safely perfused by a single perforating vessel [421], giving the anatomical basis to build two separate skin paddles not only by de-epithelization [110], but also by complete transection of the flap between both perforators. To facilitate identification of the perforators, preoperative mapping using an audible Doppler is strongly advised. Direct closure of the skin is achieved up to a flap width of 6–7 cm in the upper and middle third of the lower leg, whereas distally, skin grafts have to be used for wound coverage in the most cases. After flap raising, the patient is immobilized for 3–4 days and then allowed to ambulate with physiotherapeutic assistance.

Advantages and Disadvantages

The fibula is the longest bone flap available and can be transferred as a bone flap or in combination with one or two skin paddles. Its spectrum of indications therefore reaches from bony reconstruction at the extremities to replacement of the whole mandible, including closure of large perforating defects of the oral cavity. Flap raising can be carried out using the two-team approach, making this donor site attractive especially for primary reconstructions in the head and neck area. The quality of the thin and pliable skin paddle is comparable to the radial forearm skin, and the 3- to 5-cm-wide septum provides good flexibility to the skin island, which can be brought into the oral cavity for lining without tension. Thus, the osteocutaneous fibula flap is perfectly suited for reconstruction of composite defects of the mandible. The flap possesses a sufficiently long and high-caliber vascular pedicle, making microsurgical anastomoses easy to perform. Although the vertical dimension of the fibula is limited to half of a toothed mandible, enosseous dental implants can usually be inserted, reaching a high primary stability due to the high amount of cortical bone. The limited height of the fibula is not a problem in patients who already have atrophy of the alveolar process because there are no considerable differences in the height between the fibula and the atrophied mandible. In nonatrophied, toothed mandibles, the double-fibula transplant was suggested to compensate for the narrowness of the transplant in order to create better prerequisites for prosthetic management. The majority of authors were able to show, however, that prosthetic rehabilitation is also possible without using a double transplant [153, 172, 227, 418]. However, thinning of the skin flap around the implant is always necessary before prosthetic rehabilitation can be initiated. Despite the numerous advantages attributed to skin quality, bone length, and vascular pedicle, for isolated bone defects of the mandible not exceeding the midline, the iliac crest should be preferred because it is better suited to mimicking the natural shape of the lower jaw. The frequency of arteriosclerotic changes in the lower leg vessels is a well-known clinical fact and must be taken into consideration in the choice of flaps. Although some authors [91, 153, 234] considered that a routine angiography in cases of clinically normal findings at the foot pulses was not justified, the majority of authors assess the donor site's vascular anatomy and the vascular integrity using preoperative measures such as angiography or magnetic resonance tomography (MRT) [225, 243, 382, 431, 447]. Clinical experience shows that one out of five candidates has to be excluded from fibula transfer due to severe arteriosclerotic damage or venous insufficiency of the lower leg vessels [431]. The reliability of skin supply was another criticism of the osteocutaneous fibula transplant and has been the reason for numerous studies in which particularly the variability of the cutaneous perforating vessels and the limited size of the skin island have been reported as disadvantageous [51, 110, 152, 153, 172, 343, 418, 445]. According to the reports by Hidalgo [154] and Schusterman [343], a loss of the skin island must be considered in 7–9% of cases. Based on the anatomical studies and clinical experience of other authors [177, 399, 416, 418, 421, 425, 431], the transition of the middle and distal third of the fibula is a reliable donor site for the fibula skin paddle, which at this location is supplied by septocutaneous peroneal perforators. Having a survival rate of at least 95%, the safety of this skin paddle does not differ from other proven transplants [177, 399, 418, 431]. The possibility of forming two isolated skin islands, which was already demonstrated by Yoshimura, extends its indications [447]. Nevertheless, Yokoo and co-workers pointed out that the perforator of the skin paddle as a variation can branch off from the tibialis posterior instead from the peroneal vessels [444]. In these cases, it is necessary to directly anastomose the perforating vessel or, if no other peroneal cutaneous perforator is available, to use a second skin flap. A neurocutaneous reinnervation by connecting the sural nerve, as suggested by Sadove et al. [324] and Wei et al. [418], is not an absolute requirement for sensory innervation of the flap; rather, it seems in at least some cases that there is spontaneous neurocutaneous reinnervation due to sprouting of sensory fibers from the periphery. Some authors report the length of the vascular pedicle as ranging from 4 to a maximum of 8 cm so that in many of their cases vein grafts were necessary [110, 227, 406]. The dissectible vascular pedicle length is, however, much longer, if the transplant is raised from the distal third of the lower leg, where not only the skin supply is more reliable via septocutaneous perforating vessels, but where the fibula is better perfused via periosteal branches [425]. Vein grafts may only become necessary if long bone segments are required for subtotal mandible reconstruction because in these cases, proximal lengthening by separation from the fibula is only possible to a limited extent. A short vascular pedicle can also result if the exit of the peroneal artery lies more distally, which can, however, be recognized preoperatively by angiography.

The literature reports that donor site morbidity of the fibula flap is generally low. Apart from hypesthesia at the lateral malleolus, slight initial pain and a tendency toward edema can be found, and the flexing or stretching function of the large toe or ankle joint is objectively reduced but hardly perceived subjectively [79, 124, 153]. Nevertheless, some patients report pain and weakness on ambulation for several months after surgery [38, 257, 399], and a lower preferred velocity on walking was found compared with control subjects [38]. Instability of the ankle joint was not found in any of the patients [79, 220]. Development of radiological signs of osteoporosis can occur in the distal fibula segment after several years, but not leading to any disability on ambulation or shape of the ankle joint [220]. Hematomas can occur because of oozing from the resection margins of the bone at the donor site, and care must be taken to prevent development of a compartment syndrome [74]. Primary closure of the donor site defect should only be undertaken if this can be accomplished with no tension, because according to a study of Shindo et al., primary closure otherwise tends to a higher rate of complications compared with split-thickness skin grafting [355]. In order to ensure optimal healing of split-thickness skin grafts, a tie-over dressing should be applied and the lower leg should be immobilized for about 3–4 days.

Flap Raising

Preoperative Management

Because of possible variations of the tibial posterior and anterior vessels and the prevalence of arteriosclerotic damage in the lower extremities, conventional angiography or, less invasive, magnetic resonance angiography is mandatory before raising the fibula flap. Patients showing clinical signs of vascular damage (varicosis, missing foot pulses, pain on ambulation) should primarily be excluded. Marking the cutaneous perforators along the posterior intermuscular septum using a Doppler facilitates intraoperative exposure of these vessels.

Patient Positioning

The leg is bent into the knee joint and brought in a lateral decubitus position to obtain better access to the lateral and posterior aspect of the calf. This is facilitated by supporting the hip with a beanbag. The entire lower extremity is prepped circumferentially, and the foot is draped, leaving the pulses accessible. No tourniquet is used, because identification of the pulsating perforators is easier in the perfused leg. With consequent hemostasis and careful dissection, flap raising is possible without any significant bleeding, and the risk for diffuse oozing after release of the tourniquet and postoperative hematoma formation (compartment phenomenon) is reduced.

Flap Design

Although mapping the perforators and thus positioning the skin island is possible preoperatively using a Doppler, the skin paddle should not be designed until the cutaneous branches are clearly seen intraoperatively. In the standard situation, the skin paddle is centered vertically along the septum with its center at the junction between the middle and lower third of the fibula. If only one perforator is enclosed, the flap size should not exceed 6×10 cm. A distance of 8 cm from the lower osteotomy to the ankle must be maintained for stability of the malleolar joint; proximally, a 6-cm bone segment is maintained to protect the peroneal nerve.

Skin incision is made along the peroneus longus muscle, keeping a distance of 2 cm to the posterior intermuscular septum, which can easily be palpated posterior to the muscle. According to the location of the perforator found by preoperative mapping, the incision is slightly curved anteriorly in the region of the skin paddle. The strong crural fascia is incised following the skin incision.

`Step 1`

The perforator is visualized by carefully separating the fascia from the peroneal muscles and blunt dissection in the posterior direction. The posterior intermuscular septum, which covers the perforator from both sides, is exposed and must always be left intact in the region of the osteocutaneous flap. Once the perforator is identified, the peroneal muscles are retracted anteriorly, and the lateral margin of fibula is palpated.

`Step 2`

Proximal to the skin paddle, the posterior intermuscular septum is incised sharply along the lateral margin of the fibula. To obtain better access to the deep flexor space, the peroneal muscles are retracted anteriorly and the soleus muscle is retracted posteriorly using sharp hooks. Dorsal to the fibula bone, the flexor hallucis longus muscle becomes visible.

`Step 3`

The strong attachment of the flexor hallucis muscle to the fibula is divided carefully with scissors proximal to the skin paddle. Care must be taken not to enter too deeply into the deep flexor space, where the peroneal vessels are located.

`Step 4`

Step 5   After transecting the attachment of the flexor hallucis longus muscle to the fibula and opening the deep flexor space, the muscles can be retracted easily, and the muscular branches of the peroneal vessels are exposed.

Step 6   Continuing the dissection into the deep flexor space and tracing the muscular branches in a proximal direction, the peroneal vessels are identified. Dissection must be performed carefully to prevent any bleeding from the peroneal vessels. In the perfused leg, the artery can easily be palpated at the posterior aspect of the fibula. A number of small vessels branch off from the peroneal artery to the surrounding muscles and the fibula bone.

Step 7   A vessel loop is placed around the peroneal vessels, and the branches to the surrounding muscles and the fibular bone are clipped and transected. Perfusion of the distal bone segment is maintained and remains reliable despite the sacrifice of the proximal bone feeders. Dissection of the pedicle is facilitated by complete relaxation of the patient and plantar flexion of the foot to reduce tension of the flexor muscles.

Step 8   The peroneal muscles are retracted anteriorly, leaving a small cuff of muscle around the perforator, and a curved raspatory is positioned subperiosteally around the fibula to protect the distal peroneal vessels. The distal osteotomy is now performed with an oscillating saw, keeping a distance of 8 cm from the ankle.

Step 9   The proximal osteotomy is carried out in the same fashion. The longer the bone segment needed for reconstruction, the shorter the vascular pedicle will become. In the standard situation, at least 10 cm of pedicle length is obtained using this technique.

Step 10   The anterior intermuscular septum is incised between both osteotomies directly at the anterior rim of the fibula. The periosteum is left untouched along the whole length of the bone segment.

Step 11   The extensor muscles are bluntly separated from the fibular bone epiperiosteally, until the interosseous membrane is reached. The tibial anterior vessels are located medially underneath the extensor muscles and should not be exposed.

Step 12   The interosseous membrane is completely divided, keeping a distance of 1 cm from the fibula, and the fibers of the tibialis posterior muscle become visible. Small bleedings, originating from muscular perforators of the peroneal vessels, are carefully cauterized.

Step 13   After the interosseous membrane has been completely divided, the bone segment can be retracted laterally, and the peroneal vessels are exposed by bluntly separating the fibers of the tibialis posterior muscle at the distal osteotomy. The vessels are ligated and transected distally.

The tibialis posterior muscle is divided where the V-like fibers meet at the midline, so that a cuff of the muscle is left attached to the fibula bone segment. The flexor hallucis longus muscle and the posterior intermuscular septum are left untouched.

Step 14

To obtain access to the flexor hallucis longus muscle from both sides, the skin paddle now is peritomized to the level of the crural fascia, which is included in the skin paddle to safely protect the perforating vessel. The fascia is transected using scissors, keeping a safe distance from the cutaneous vessel.

Step 15

The bone, skin paddle, and the posterior intermuscular septum are elevated, and a cuff of soleus muscle is left attached to the septum around the perforator during separation of the skin paddle from the underlying muscles.

Step 16

Keeping a distance of at least 2 cm from the bone, the flexor hallucis longus muscle and the posterior intermuscular septum are transected, and the flap can now be moved laterally. The peroneal vessels are completely covered by the muscle cuff, built by the tibialis posterior and flexor muscles. The cutaneous perforator is seen in the middle of the posterior intermuscular septum.

Step 17

At the proximal osteotomy, fibers of the flexor hallucis muscle are transected by carefully retracting the vascular pedicle.

Step 18

The flap is now ready for microvascular transfer. A longer pedicle can be obtained by further dissection of the peroneal vessels up to the level of the bifurcation with the tibial posterior vessels, but this is only necessary if a long bone segment is needed for reconstruction. Direct wound closure is achieved if the width of the skin flap does not exceed 2 cm; in all other cases, a split-thickness skin graft is used for covering the donor site defect. A deep drain is inserted, and the soleus and peroneus muscles are loosely attached to form a well-vascularized bed for the skin graft. The patient normally is immobilized for 3–4 days and then is allowed to ambulate with physiotherapeutic assistance. Foot pulses are controlled regularly during the first 24 h.

Step 19

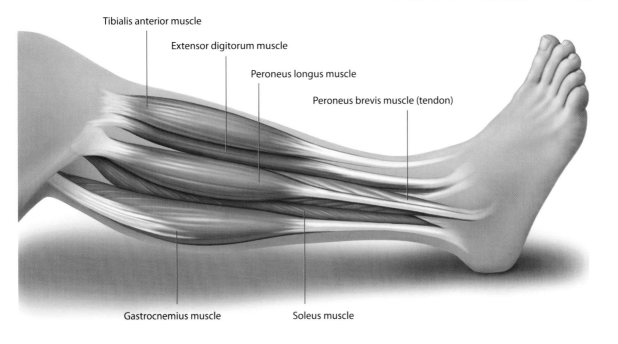

Tibialis anterior muscle

Extensor digitorum muscle

Peroneus longus muscle

Peroneus brevis muscle (tendon)

Gastrocnemius muscle

Soleus muscle

Muscles of the lateral lower leg

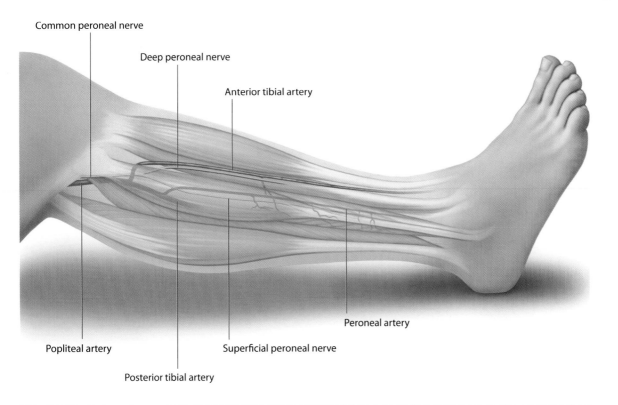

Common peroneal nerve

Deep peroneal nerve

Anterior tibial artery

Peroneal artery

Popliteal artery

Superficial peroneal nerve

Posterior tibial artery

Arteries of the lower leg

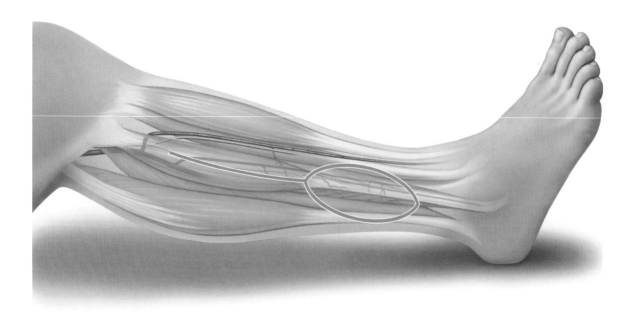

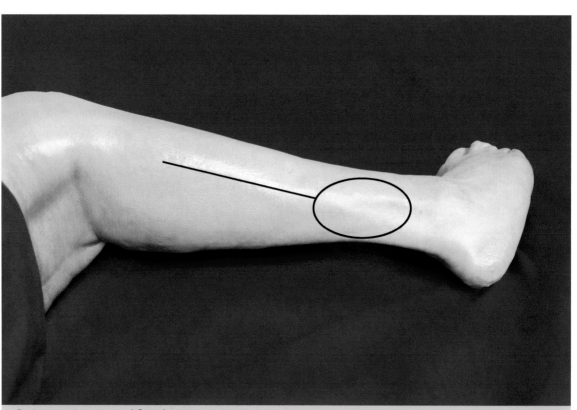

Patient positioning and flap design

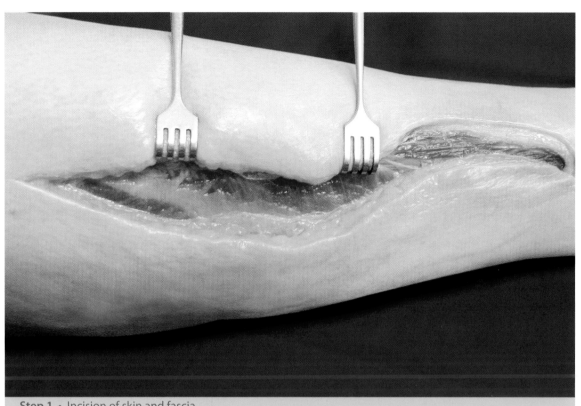

Step 1 • Incision of skin and fascia

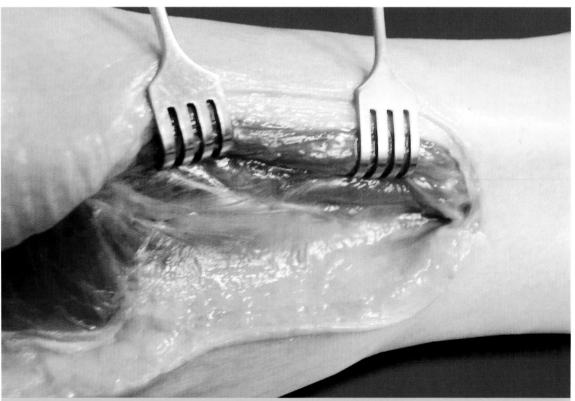

Step 2 • Identification of perforator

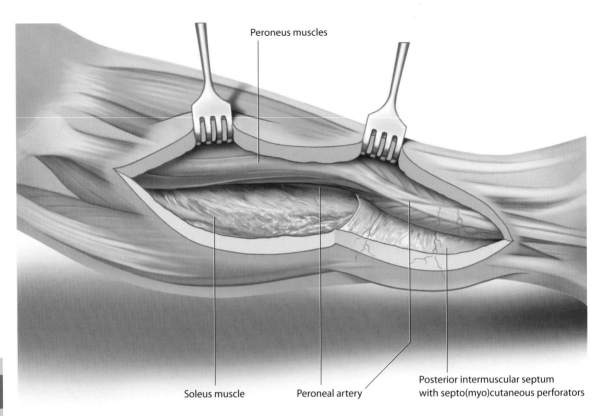

Peroneus muscles

Soleus muscle   Peroneal artery   Posterior intermuscular septum
                                                            with septo(myo)cutaneous perforators

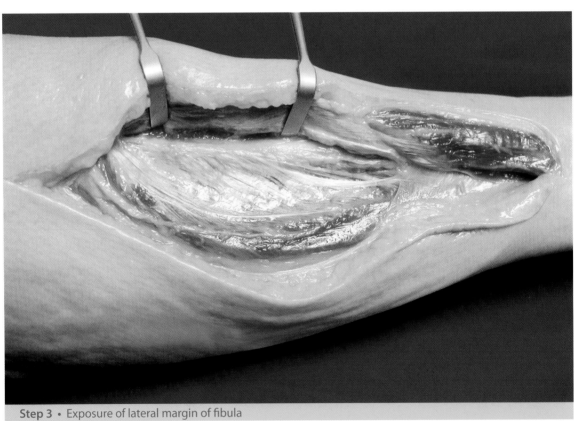

Step 3 • Exposure of lateral margin of fibula

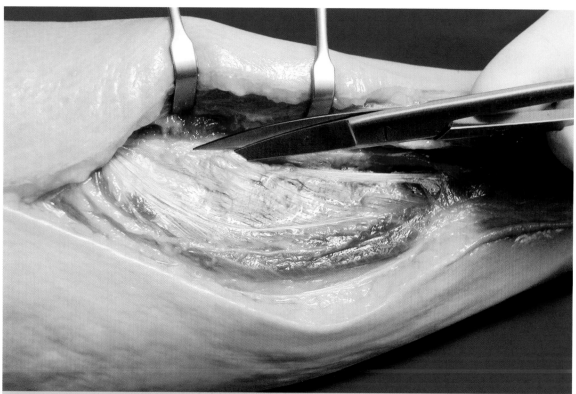

Step 4 • Detachment of soleus and flexor hallucis longus muscle

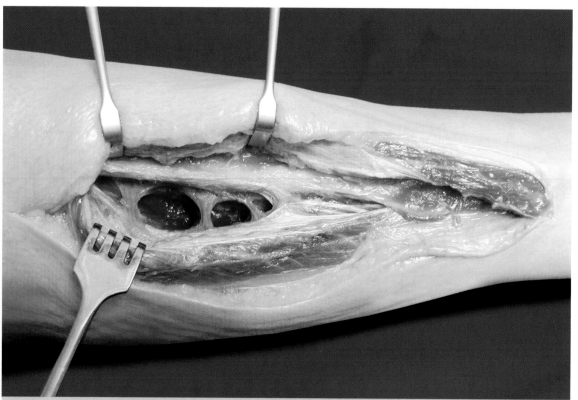

Step 5 • Opening of deep flexor space, identification of peroneal branches

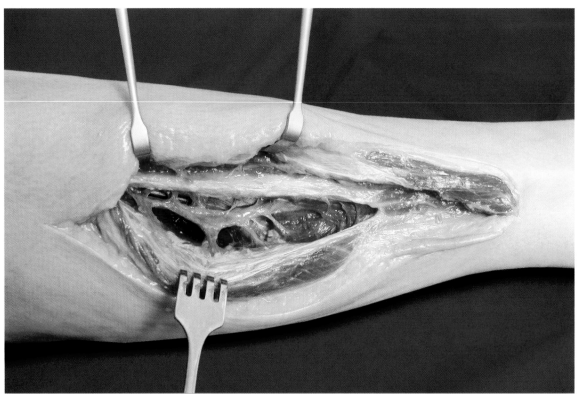

Step 6 • Exposure of peroneal vessels

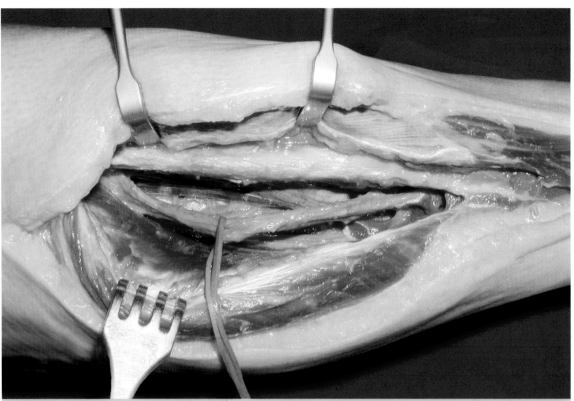

Step 7 • Dissection of vascular pedicle

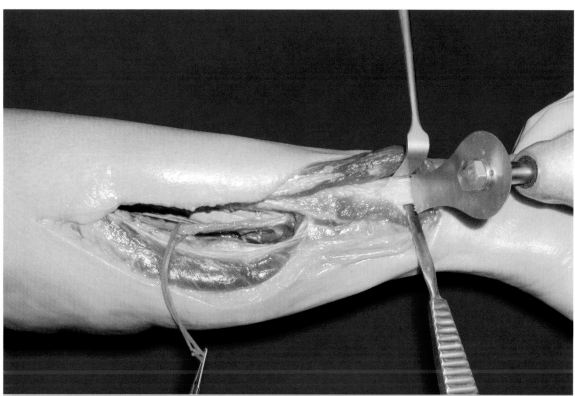

Step 8 • Distal osteotomy

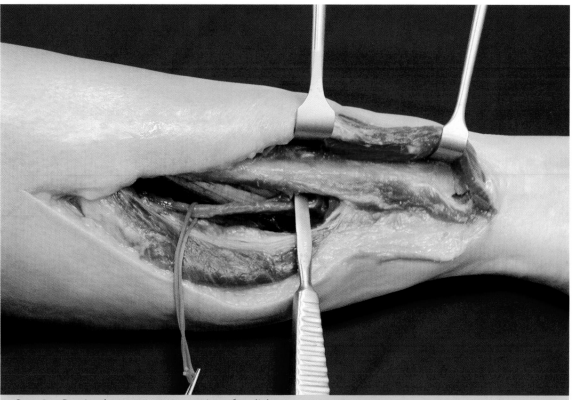

Step 9 • Proximal osteotomy, protection of pedicle

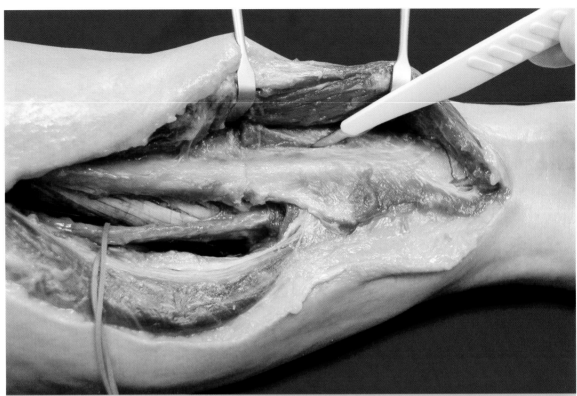

Step 10 • Incision of anterior intermuscular septum

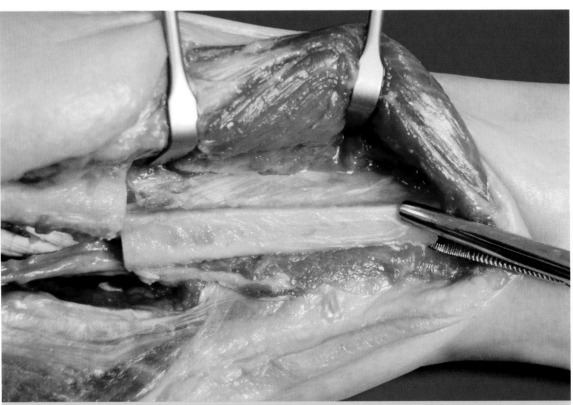

Step 11 • Exposure of interosseous membrane

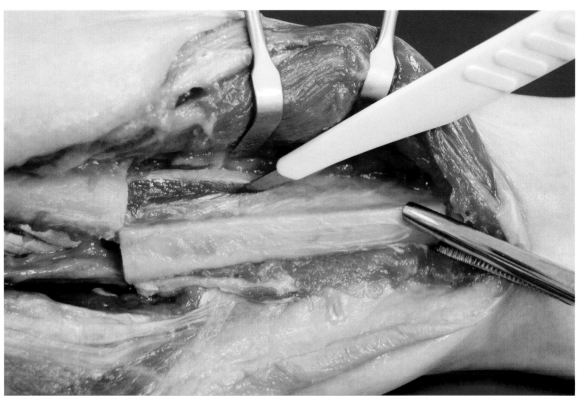

Step 12 • Transection of interosseous membrane

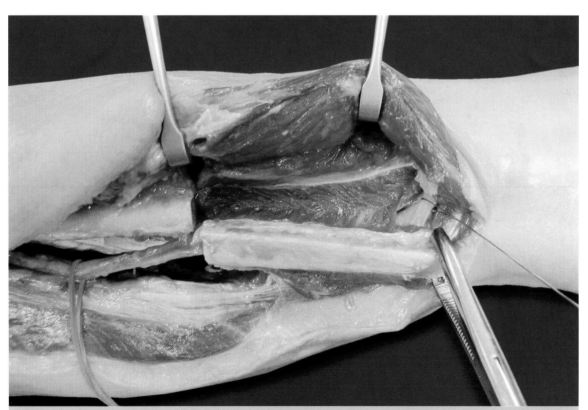

Step 13 • Distal ligation of peroneal vessels

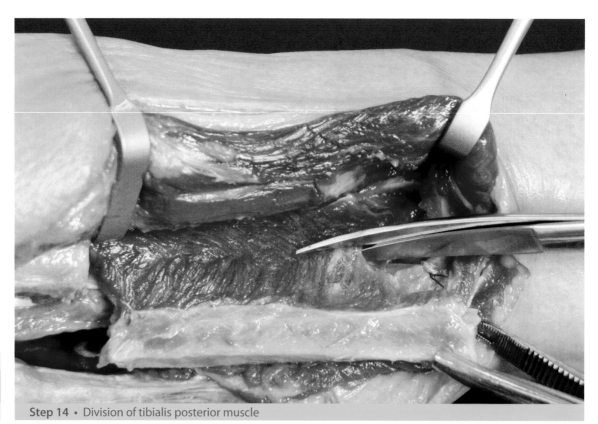

Step 14 • Division of tibialis posterior muscle

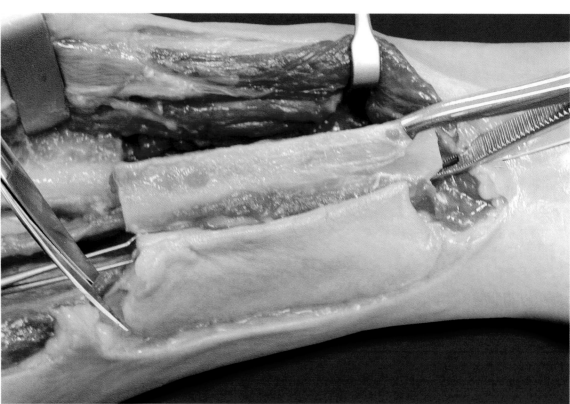

Step 15 • Incision of skin and fascia at dorsal periphery of skin paddle

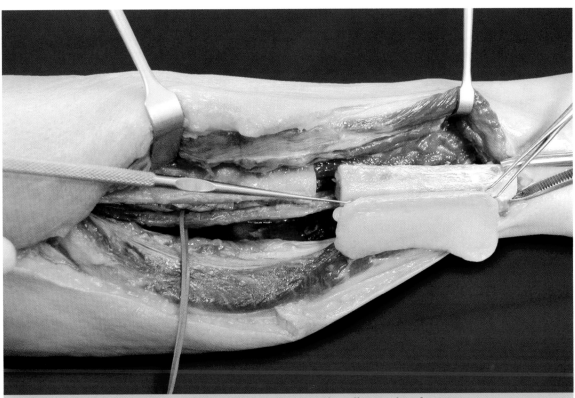

Step 16 • Complete elevation of skin paddle including muscle cuff around perforator

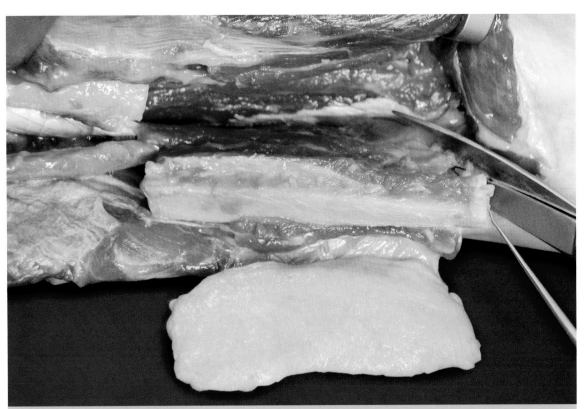

Step 17 • Distal transection of flexor hallucis longus muscle

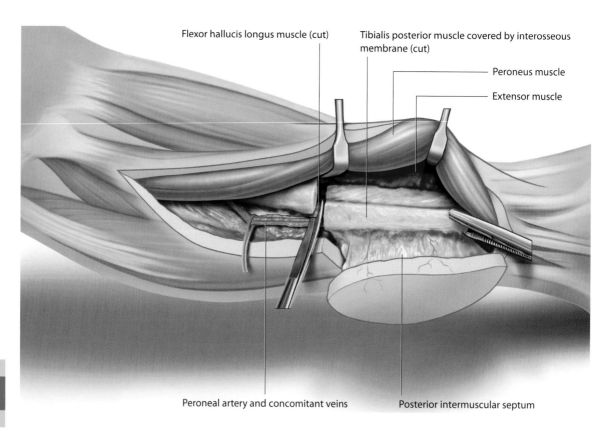

Flexor hallucis longus muscle (cut)

Tibialis posterior muscle covered by interosseous membrane (cut)

Peroneus muscle

Extensor muscle

Peroneal artery and concomitant veins

Posterior intermuscular septum

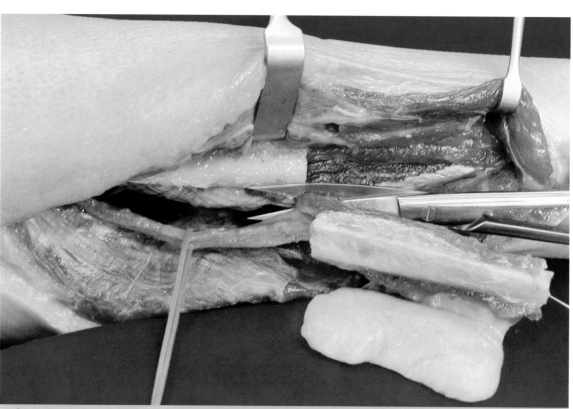

Step 18 • Proximal transection of remaining flexor hallucis muscle fibers

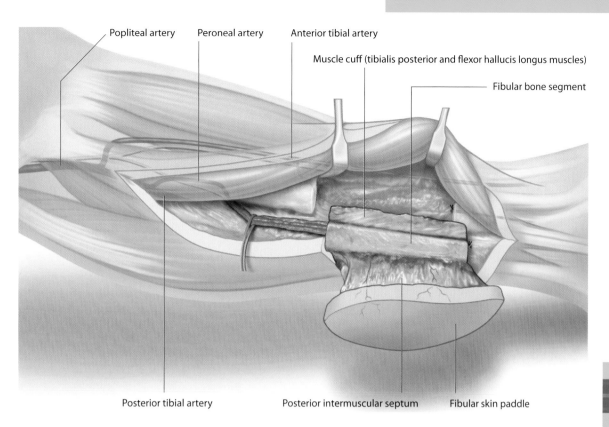

Popliteal artery   Peroneal artery   Anterior tibial artery

Muscle cuff (tibialis posterior and flexor hallucis longus muscles)

Fibular bone segment

Posterior tibial artery   Posterior intermuscular septum   Fibular skin paddle

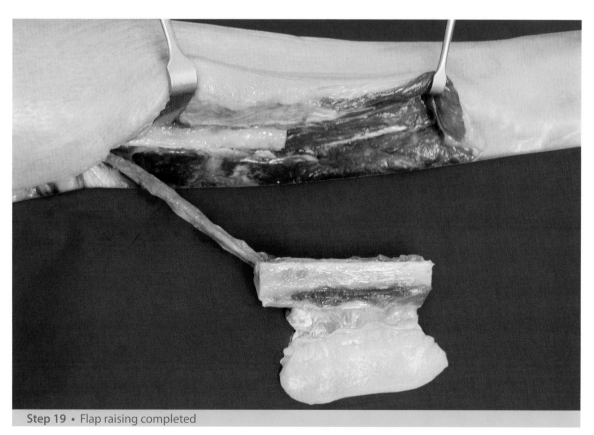

Step 19 • Flap raising completed

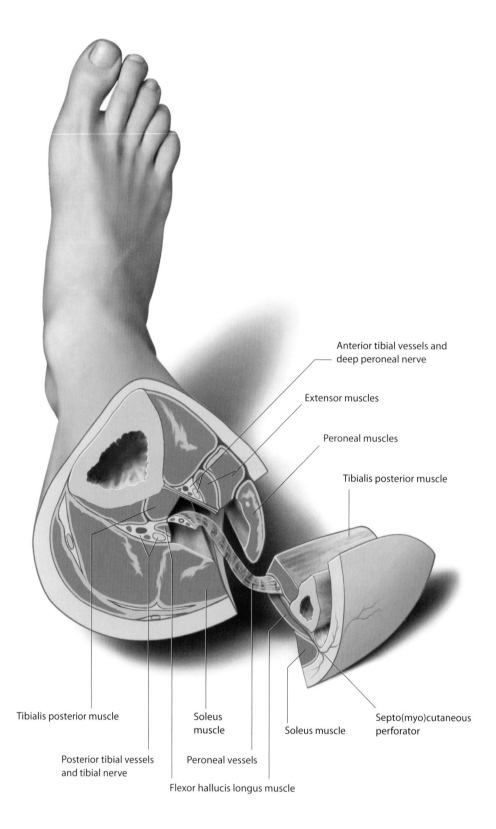

Anterior tibial vessels and
deep peroneal nerve

Extensor muscles

Peroneal muscles

Tibialis posterior muscle

Tibialis posterior muscle

Soleus
muscle

Soleus muscle

Septo(myo)cutaneous
perforator

Posterior tibial vessels
and tibial nerve

Peroneal vessels

Flexor hallucis longus muscle

Cross-section anatomy of the osteocutaneous fibular flap and donor site

Comments

Flap Design

The posterior intermuscular septum is the key structure in designing the skin paddle. Sometimes it is mistaken with the anterior intermuscular septum, which is located between the peroneus and the extensor muscles. The posterior intermuscular septum can easily be identified by palpating the groove between the Achilles tendon and peroneus muscles above the ankle, which then can be followed proximally.

Step 2: If no perforator is found at the transition of the middle and distal third of the lower leg, the whole septum has to be inspected, and another perforator is selected at the proximal calf. If no appropriate perforator can be identified along the whole septum, the contralateral leg should be considered for flap raising. This situation occurs in about 1% of all cases.

Step 3: The posterior intermuscular septum may only be opened proximal to the planned bone segment and must be left intact along the entire length of the fibular bone flap and skin paddle.

Step 4: Further septo(myo)cutaneous and muscular branches can be found while opening the posterior intermuscular septum and the deep flexor space. These vessels must be carefully ligated or clipped to prevent postoperative bleeding complications.

Steps 5, 6, 7: Exposure and dissection of the peroneal vessels may be difficult if the patient is not positioned properly. The knee must be bent and the hip must be elevated for easy access to the dorsal aspect of the lower leg. During blunt separation of the muscle fibers, one of the comitant veins becomes visible first. Always control the location of the peroneal artery by palpating the peroneus pulse.

Step 8: The cutaneous perforator regularly sends a branch to the peroneal muscles, so that bleeding will occur when forming the muscle cuff. Keep a distance of about 1 cm from the cutaneous branch to be able to cauterize the muscle bleeding without damaging the skin vessel.

Steps 8, 9: Be sure that the posterior intermuscular septum remains intact along the entire length of the osteotomized fibula segment. This will guarantee the protection of the septocutaneous vessel and the attachment of the skin paddle to the bone.

Steps 10, 12: For incision of the anterior intermuscular septum and the interosseous membrane, use a sharp scalpel and do not violate the underlying muscles.

Step 13: Expose the distal tibial posterior vessels carefully to prevent bleeding from the veins and to be able to make a safe ligation.

Step 14: During transection of the tibialis posterior muscle, bleeding will occur from the connecting branches to the tibial posterior artery and branches to the surrounding muscles. Carefully clip or cauterize these vessels.

Step 15: The sural nerve and posterior saphenous vein may become exposed at the dorsal periphery of the skin flap and might be ligated, if necessary.

Step 16: To facilitate elevation of the flap, hold the skin paddle between two fingers to protect the septum and the cutaneous vessel from both sides. Leave a cuff of soleus muscle along the whole length of the septum, with its greatest thickness of about 1 cm around the perforator.

Step 17: When the posterior intermuscular septum, which is still fixated to the tibial bone, is transected medial to the tibialis posterior muscle, great mobility is achieved, and the flap can now easily be moved laterally. Further medially, the tibial nerve and the tibial posterior vessels will become visible. Great care must be taken not to injure these structures.

Iliac Crest Bone Flap

Wolff/Hölzle, *Raising of Microvascular Flaps 2nd ed.*,
DOI: 10.1007/978-3-642-13831-7_7, © Springer-Verlag Berlin Heidelberg 2011

Development and Indications

The transfer of bone blocks of the ileum as parts of composite flaps from the groin donor site was described in anatomical studies by Taylor and Watson in 1978 [383]. These authors used this flap pedicled on the superficial circumflex iliac artery (SCIA) for reconstruction of compound defects of the lower leg. Whereas the blood supply of the SCIA was excellent to the skin, the bone blocks of the iliac crest were only perfused marginally by these vessels. Other vascular pedicles around the hip, such as the ascending branch of the circumflex femoral artery or the superior gluteal artery, were also used for microvascular transfer of composite flaps containing bone from the iliac crest [17, 163]. Although the vascular anatomy of the groin region, which was the first donor site for free flaps [11], was already investigated by Taylor and Daniel in 1973 [381], it took until 1979, when Taylor et al. [383] and Sanders and Mayou [329] described the first transfer of the iliac crest bone, using the deep circumflex iliac artery (DCIA) as the vascular pedicle. Both groups independently identified the DCIA as the main nutrient vessel of the entire ileum. Since these first reports, the iliac crest proved to be a useful and reliable donor site, which, because of its anatomical shape, is ideally suited for the harvest of bone flaps to reconstruct defects of up to half a mandible [4, 28, 29, 85, 99, 106, 178, 179, 308, 378, 379, 401, 403]. Because of the high amount of bone available, enosseous dental implants can be inserted without problems, making the iliac crest the donor site of first choice for functional masticatory reconstruction of the mandible and maxilla [308]. Sanders and Mayou also have shown that the DCIA provides blood supply to the overlying skin of the iliac crest by myocutaneous vessels [329]; thus, a skin paddle from the groin region can additionally be included and used for extra- or intraoral reconstruction [179, 308, 401, 403]. Other flaps, such as the anterolateral thigh flap, have also been transferred together with the iliac crest [209] to extend the skin territory for soft tissue reconstruction, performing additional anastomoses at the descending branch of the circumflex femoral artery because of the bulk and the limited maneuverability of the iliac crest skin paddle. Urken and co-workers introduced the inclusion of the internal oblique muscle into the iliac osteomyocutaneous flap [399, 401, 403]. They proposed using this flat and flexible muscle for intraoral lining instead of the voluminous skin paddle. Although it was shown by Ramasastry et al. in 1984 [302] that the internal oblique muscle is safely perfused by the ascending branch of the DCIA, thus making it possible to build a vascularized myo-osseous iliac flap pedicled on the DCIA, the internal oblique muscle was only used as an isolated muscle flap until Urken's description. Apart from the decreased bulk, covering the iliac crest with the internal oblique muscle is advantageous for prosthetic rehabilitation following the insertion of enosseous dental implants. Given the secondary atrophy of the muscle, a tight and flat residual tissue, similar to that of the attached gingiva, will develop, allowing for good hygiene and loadability around the implants. The iliac crest internal oblique flap also has proven to be useful in covering skull base defects and in reconstructing the hard palate.

Anatomy

The anatomy of the DCIA was first described by Taylor et al. in detail [383]. The artery arises directly cranial (57%) to the inguinal ligament from the external iliac artery or directly caudal to it from the femoral artery (42%), mostly opposite the inferior epigastric artery [162]. The diameter of the artery varies between 1.5 and 3 mm [27, 289, 383]. Two comitant veins are usually found, which merge 1–2 cm before entering the external iliac vein; here, the vein has a caliber of 3–5 mm. Between the transversalis and iliacus fascia, the vascular pedicle courses toward the anterior superior iliac spine (ASIS), about 2 cm cranial to the connecting line between the tuberculum pubicum and the ASIS, representing the inguinal ligament. After having reached the anterior margin of the iliac crest approximately 2 cm inferior to the ASIS, the DCIA courses along the inner aspect of the ileum dorsally, located in the groove formed by the iliacus and transversus muscles. In the region of the iliosacral joint, the DCIA anastomoses with the thoracolumbar artery, which has an outer diameter of 2 mm and could also serve as the vascular pedicle if the DCIA has been transected following previous surgery [63]. During its course, the DCIA gives rise to several branches to the iliacus muscle, as well as periosteal and medullary perforators to the iliac crest. Moreover, the DCIA gives rise to the ascending branch, which runs at the undersurface of the internal oblique muscle. During its course along the inner aspect of the ileum, a number of myocutaneous perforators arise from the DCIA, piercing all three muscle layers of the abdominal wall. These three to nine fine perforators enter the skin within an approximately 2.5-cm-wide cuff of the externus oblique muscle, beginning at the ASIS and reaching about 10 cm distally. This muscle cuff always has to be incorporated when elevating a skin paddle. If the bulk of the muscle cuff needs to be reduced, a perforator-based skin paddle can be harvested, provided the exact location of the perforating vessel to the skin has been confirmed by ultrasound preoperatively [189]. Apart from the above-mentioned periosteal and medullary branches, the bone is additionally supplied by the well-perfused cuff of the iliacus and oblique muscles, which has to be left attached to the bone during flap harvesting. The results of anatomical studies and clinical experience have shown that bone flaps can include the whole iliac crest, extending from the ASIS up to the iliosacral joint [27–29, 289, 308, 329, 383, 399]. Angiographically, Taylor was able to identify a number of foramina at the iliac crest, allowing the DCIA to anastomose with branches from the inferior gluteal artery, giving the anatomical basis to include parts of the gluteus muscle in the flap [233, 286, 383]. These findings where confirmed using dye injections, which have also shown that the skin paddle supplied by the DCIA can be extended along the whole ileum, reaching close to the inferior rib arch. The most important side branch of the DCIA is the ascending branch, which mostly arises from the vascular pedicle (80%) before it reaches the ASIS [399]. In the remaining cases, multiple smaller branches can be found, which reach the undersurface of the internal oblique distally and laterally to the ASIS. Another branching pattern was described by Taylor, who found the ascending branch to arise in every third case from the proximal, interme-diate, and distal segment of the vascular pedicle between the iliac artery and the ASIS [383]. This branch, measuring 1–2 mm in diameter, pro-vides the dominant blood supply to the internal oblique muscle, but it does not contribute to skin perfusion. This branch allows for integration of nearly the entire internal oblique muscle, which can be used for intra-oral lining [99, 399, 401, 403]. Another side branch is typically found just proximal to the ASIS to reach the iliacus muscle. The lateral femoral cuta-neous nerve, which mostly crosses the DCIA superficially, provides sen-sation to the lateral and proximal aspect of the thigh. Although this cutaneous nerve can be identified medial to the ASIS and preserved by meticulous dissection, it is normally sacrificed during dissection of the pedicle, because numbness at the thigh is not negatively registered by patients. The vascular pedicle was never found to be absent [399], and in addition to the above-mentioned variations concerning the ascending branch, only the veins join at a variable distance from the external iliac vein, sometimes making two separate anastomoses necessary. Moreover, in rare cases, the DCIA can be duplicated [340, 399], so that the decision as to which of the two arteries provides reliable blood supply to the flap has to be made by temporary clamping. Because of its variable exit and high caliber, the ascending branch can be mistaken for the DCIA, espe-cially in those rare cases when the DCIA passes through the transversus muscle medially to the ASIS, so that it travels more superficially along the iliac crest [383].

Advantages and Disadvantages

Because of its extensive amount of bone and the various possibilities in designing the bone flap, the iliac crest is assumed to be the ideal donor site for mandible reconstruction; moreover, the flap has the potential of being used for other osseous defects at the maxilla, skull base, tibia, metacarpus, and many other parts of the skeleton [99, 286, 308, 340, 378, 379, 399]. To restore masticatory function, augmentations to the severely atrophied mandible have been performed using this flap, which allows for problem-free implantation of dental prostheses [308]. The anatomy of the vascular pedicle has no significant variations, and donor-site morbidity is nor-mally low, even if extensive bone flaps have been removed including the ASIS. To prevent complications at the donor site, closure has to be per-formed by an experienced surgeon. After accurate hemostasis, the iliacus muscle is attached to the transversus muscle using multiple and deep sutures, which additionally can be placed through drill holes along the cut margin of the pelvic bone. Next, the internus and externus oblique mus-cles are approximated to the tensor and gluteus muscles. Finally, the sub-cutaneous fatty tissue and the skin are closed in layers. The patient is immobilized for 3–4 days, and ambulation is begun under physiothera-peutic assistance. Nevertheless, a number of complications at the donor site are known, such as herniation (9.7%), long-lasting pain (8.4%), neu-ropathy (4.8%), and impotence (1.2%) [111]. Moreover, injury to the iliohypogastric and ilioinguinal nerves is possible, which penetrate the muscles of the abdominal wall [233].

The length of the vascular pedicle is limited to about 7 cm, sometimes making anastomosis difficult, especially after radical neck dissection. In these cases, vein grafts have to be used to lengthen the pedicle [178, 286]. Due to the voluminous skin paddle, osteomyocutaneous iliac crest flaps are often too bulky for intraoral reconstruction [286, 399]. Moreover, reliability of the skin paddle can easily be reduced by kinking, stretching, or compression of the fine myocutaneous perforators. Thus, the skin island has to be handled without any tensile or compressive forces, and it must always be designed large enough to capture a high number of myocutaneous vessels, making skin perfusion reliable. Nevertheless, venous drainage of the skin can be insufficient in up to 20% if only the deep vascular system is used [178, 179, 286]. Because of this, these and other authors emphasize the importance of performing a second venous anastomosis to the superficial venous system (superficial circumflex iliac vein, SCIV), which can be included in a large skin paddle [179, 286, 329].

Flap Raising

Patient Positioning

The patient is placed in the supine position with the buttocks on the donor site elevated by a beanbag. The operating field is prepped between the midline, posterior axillary line, lower rib arch, and upper thigh. For mandible reconstruction, the ipsilateral hip is selected if the defect involves the ramus and angle and extends to the anterior arch, and if the recipient vessels arise in the region of the angle. If a skin paddle is needed for intraoral lining, the opposite hip is selected; if the skin paddle is to be placed extraorally, the flap is raised from the ipsilateral side. Because of the constant anatomy, no preoperative measures are necessary to reveal the course of the flap vessels.

Flap Design

Bone segments up to 6–8×16–18 cm can be harvested from the whole iliac crest, keeping a safe distance from the acetabulum and iliosacral joint. For mandibular reconstruction, the ASIS is used to build the angle, extending the bone flap along the iliac crest to form the body and anterior arch. The anterior border of the pelvis between the ASIS and the inferior spine is used to form the ramus of the new hemimandible. Even if the angle is not involved, inclusion of the ASIS will facilitate flap raising and does not negatively affect the appearance or morbidity of the donor site. Elliptic skin islands are outlined along the curvature of the iliac crest with the axis running 2.5 cm parallel and medial to the iliac crest. Skin islands must always be large enough to include all perforators in a zone between the ASIS and approximately 10 cm posterior to the ASIS. To raise a myo-osseous flap without a skin paddle, the incision is outlined 2 cm superior to the connection of the pubic tubercle and the ASIS, starting just lateral to the pulse of the femoral artery. For further exposure of the pelvic bone, the incision is drawn directly above the curvature of the iliac crest far enough distally to allow for easy detachment of the soft tissues.

First, skin and subcutaneous fatty tissue are incised between the femoral artery and the ASIS, and the inguinal ligament is identified. The superficial epigastric vessels may run across the incision line and are ligated and divided.

Step 1

The inguinal ligament, which forms the aponeurosis of the external iliac muscle, is incised parallel to the orientation of the ligament fibers, and the internal oblique muscle readily becomes visible. The orientation of this muscle is perpendicular to the fibers of the inguinal ligament. For the next step, the skin and ligament are retracted in a cranial direction.

Step 2

The internal oblique muscle is transected with scissors 2 cm superior to the connection of the ASIS and the pubic tubercle, and loose fatty tissue becomes visible, covering the thin transversalis fascia. The pulse of the DCIA is easily palpated in the groove formed by the transversus and iliacus muscle, and the vascular pedicle is exposed by careful and mostly blunt separation of the fatty tissue. It is not necessary to expose the external iliac artery for identification of the DCIA.

Step 3

A vessel loop is placed around the artery, which is accompanied by two veins, and the pedicle is dissected free along its course to the ASIS. Few branches to the surrounding muscles must be clipped or ligated. The ascending branch, which courses along the undersurface of the internal oblique muscle, is identified. If the lateral femoral cutaneous nerve crosses above the vascular pedicle, it is transected as well.

Step 4

Once the vascular pedicle has been isolated just medial to the ASIS, the skin incision is continued along the iliac crest to the level of the external oblique muscle.

Step 5

The lateral rim of the iliac crest is palpated, and the muscles are now transected at the gluteal aspect of the pelvis. Consequent hemostasis has to be performed to prevent diffuse bleeding from the well-perfused muscles.

Step 6

Beginning anteriorly, the tensor fasciae latae and gluteus medius muscles are detached epiperiosteally from the external surface of the hip, while the sartorius muscle is left intact. Again, careful hemostasis is necessary. The muscles of the abdominal wall are retracted in a cranial direction and bluntly undermined medial to the iliac crest, keeping a dissection plane superficial to the vascular pedicle.

Step 7

Step 8   Keeping a distance of 2 cm from the inner rim of the iliac crest, the abdominal muscles are transected with scissors from a caudal to cranial direction, and further muscular branches to the internal oblique muscle are cauterized or ligated. The pulse of the DCIA is palpated at the inner surface of the pelvic curvature 1–3 cm inferior to the inner rim and therefore can easily be preserved during transection of the muscles. A broad abdominal hook is inserted to protect and retract the content of the peritoneum. Superficial to the iliacus muscle, a thin layer of loose fatty tissue again becomes visible.

Step 9   The course of the DCIA is palpated in the groove formed by the transversus and iliacus muscle, and the iliacus muscle is sharply transected to the periosteum about 1–2 cm below the artery.

Step 10   Muscular detachment is continued at the ASIS, where the sartorius muscle is transected directly at its origin from the bone. The vascular pedicle, which is enveloped into the fascia between the iliacus and transversus muscle, must be carefully protected in the region of the ASIS while transecting the muscles.

Step 11   Osteotomy begins distally at the iliac crest after transection of the abdominal muscles covering the bone. The oscillating saw cuts through the inner and outer cortical bone until the desired depth of the bone segment is reached. Doing this, the soft tissues are retracted with broad hooks to protect the peritoneum and to visualize the blade during the osteotomy. The vascular pedicle is transected and ligated at the distal osteotomy.

Step 12   Osteotomy is continued by cutting the bone bicortically in an anterior direction, keeping a parallel distance from the upper rim of the iliac crest. The oscillating saw is inserted caudal enough at the lateral aspect of the pelvis so that the vascular pedicle cannot be injured while penetrating the inner cortical layer. If a mandibular angle and ramus has to be built, the osteotomy is continued parallel to the anterior rim of the pelvis up to a depth of 6–8 cm. Again, the vascular pedicle must be carefully protected during osteotomy.

Step 13   The osteotomized bone segment is elevated and the residual muscle fibers are transected. The vascular pedicle is dissected medially close to the external iliac vessels, the ascending branch is transected, and the artery is separated from the accompanying veins. The veins normally fuse 1–2 cm laterally to the external iliac vein.

Step 14   Perfusion of the flap is maintained until the recipient vessels are ready for anastomosis. Wound closure has to be performed by an experienced surgeon after insertion of a deep drain and accurate hemostasis. Bone wax may be used at the cutting surfaces of the pelvic bone. First, the iliacus muscle is attached to the transversus muscle using multiple and deep sutures, which additionally can be placed through drill holes along the cut margin of the pelvic bone. Next, the internal and external oblique muscles are approximated to the tensor and gluteus muscles. Finally, the subcutaneous fatty tissue and the skin are closed in layers. The patient is immobilized for 3–4 days, and ambulation is then begun under physiotherapeutic assistance.

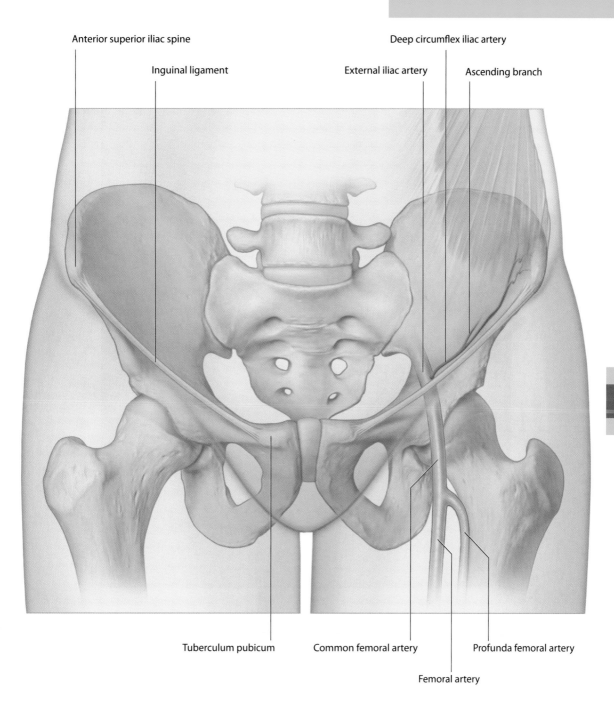

Anterior superior iliac spine

Inguinal ligament

Deep circumflex iliac artery

External iliac artery

Ascending branch

Tuberculum pubicum

Common femoral artery

Profunda femoral artery

Femoral artery

Deep circumflex iliac artery (DCIA) running along the inguinal ligament toward the inner lip of the iliac crest

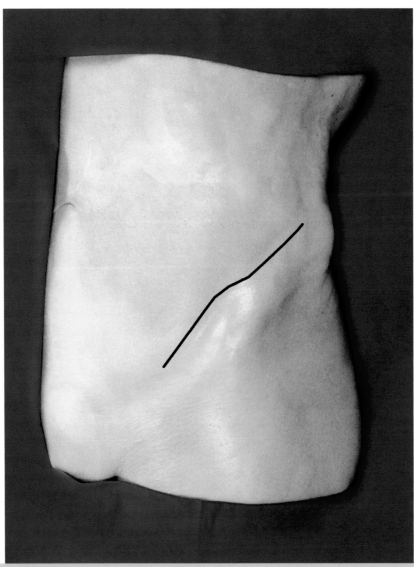

Orientation of skin incision for raising of myo-osseous iliac crest bone flaps

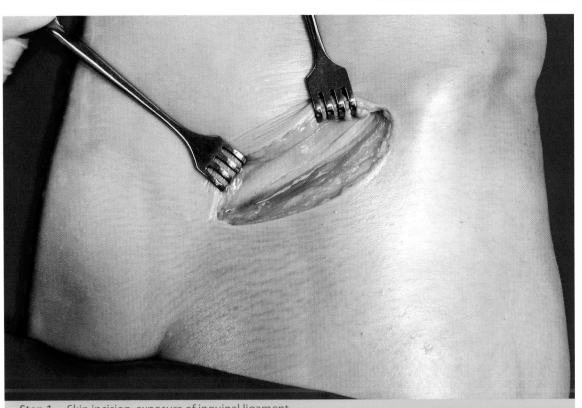

Step 1 • Skin incision, exposure of inguinal ligament

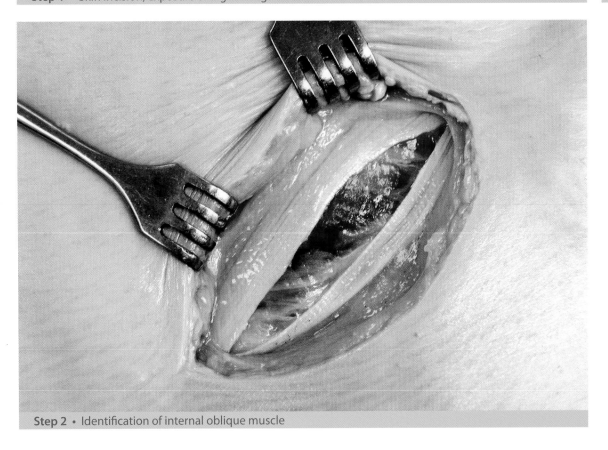

Step 2 • Identification of internal oblique muscle

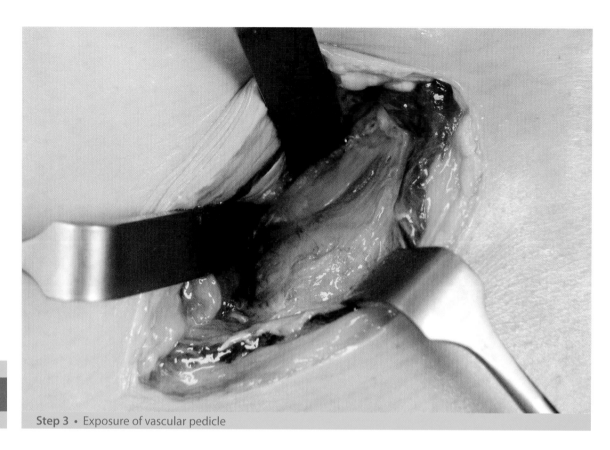

142

Step 3 • Exposure of vascular pedicle

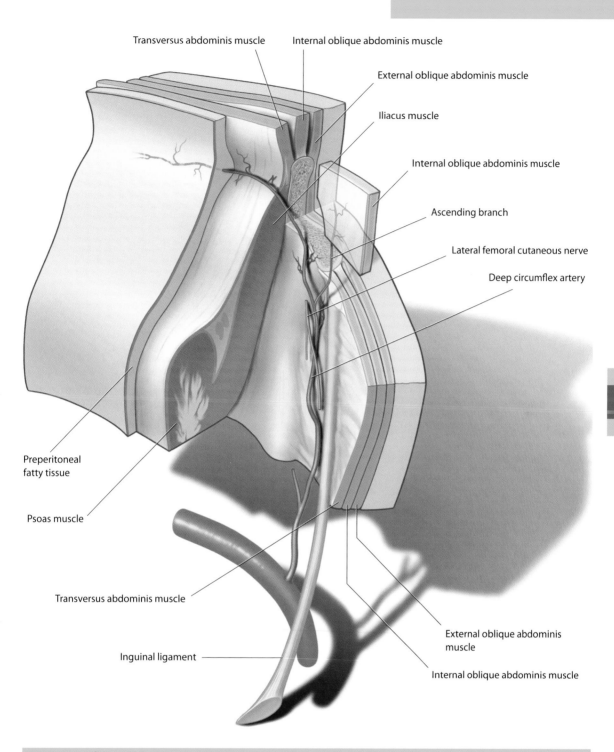

Transversus abdominis muscle

Internal oblique abdominis muscle

External oblique abdominis muscle

Iliacus muscle

Internal oblique abdominis muscle

Ascending branch

Lateral femoral cutaneous nerve

Deep circumflex artery

Preperitoneal fatty tissue

Psoas muscle

Transversus abdominis muscle

Inguinal ligament

External oblique abdominis muscle

Internal oblique abdominis muscle

Anatomy of the DCIA

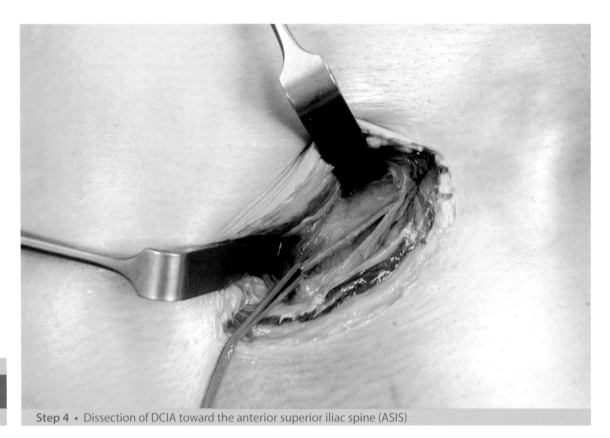

144

Step 4 • Dissection of DCIA toward the anterior superior iliac spine (ASIS)

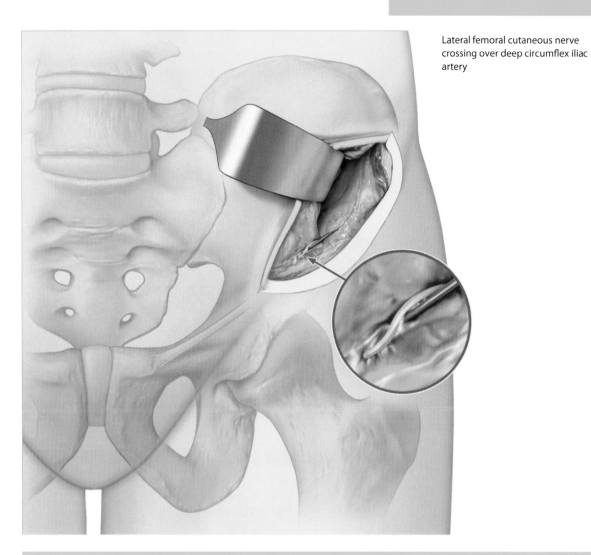

Lateral femoral cutaneous nerve crossing over deep circumflex iliac artery

Deep circumflex iliac artery

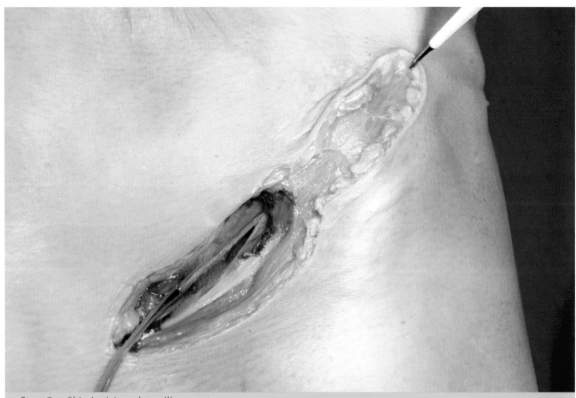

Step 5 • Skin incision along iliac crest

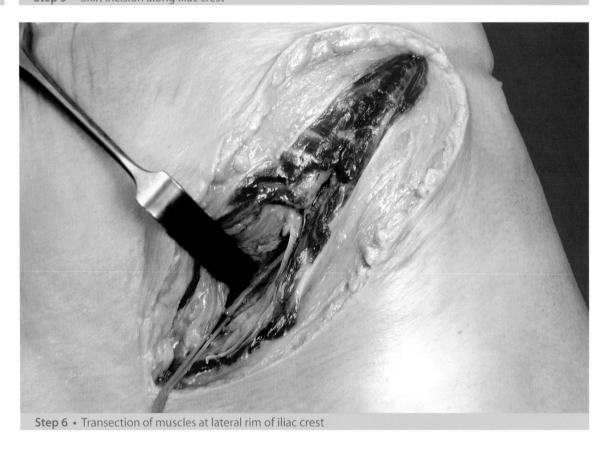

Step 6 • Transection of muscles at lateral rim of iliac crest

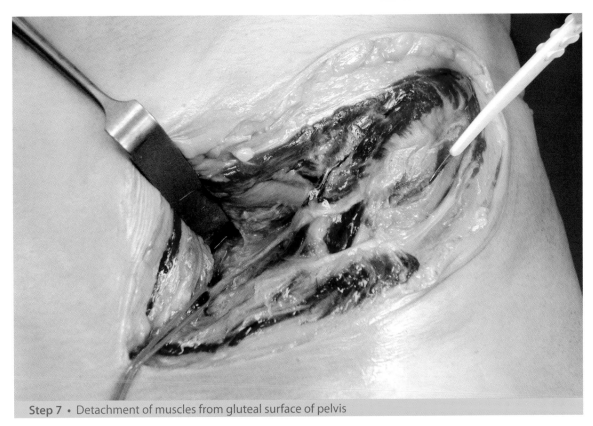

Step 7 • Detachment of muscles from gluteal surface of pelvis

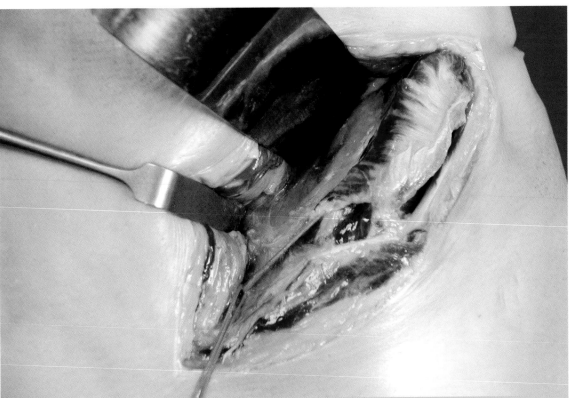

Step 8 • Transection of oblique abdominal muscles, exposure of iliacus muscle by retracting the peritoneum

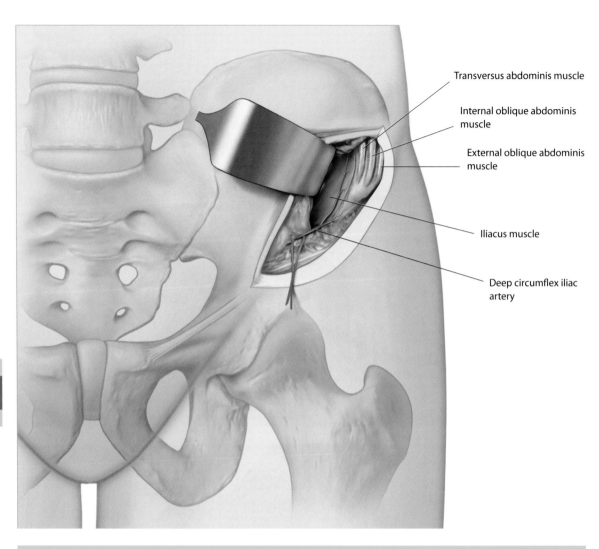

Transversus abdominis muscle

Internal oblique abdominis muscle

External oblique abdominis muscle

Iliacus muscle

Deep circumflex iliac artery

Exposure of inner aspect of pelvis showing the pedicle and iliacus muscle

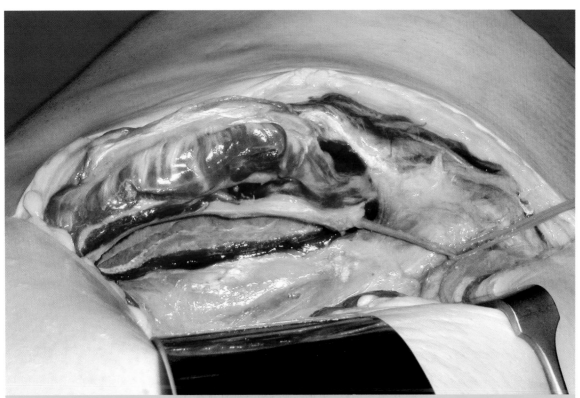

Step 9 • Incision of iliacus muscle below DCIA

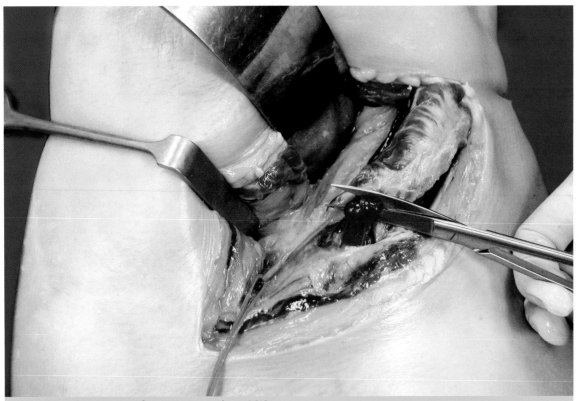

Step 10 • Transection of sartorius muscle at ASIS

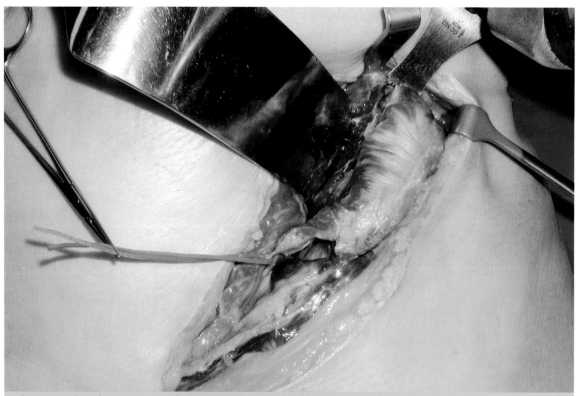

Step 11 • Distal osteotomy at iliac crest

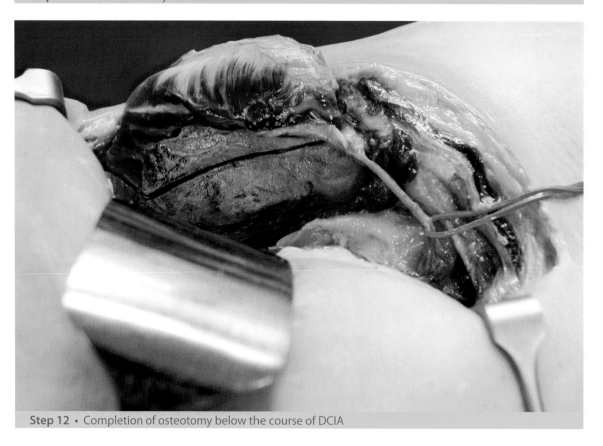

Step 12 • Completion of osteotomy below the course of DCIA

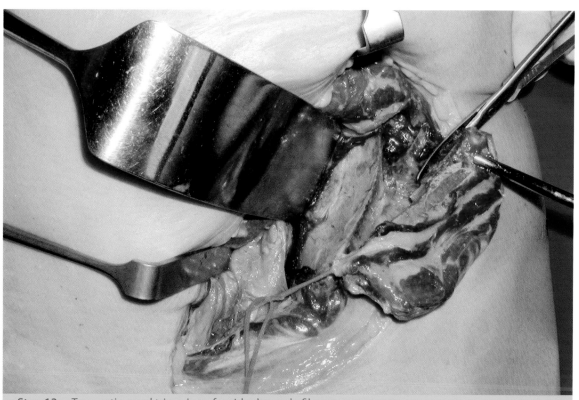

Step 13 • Transection and trimming of residual muscle fibers

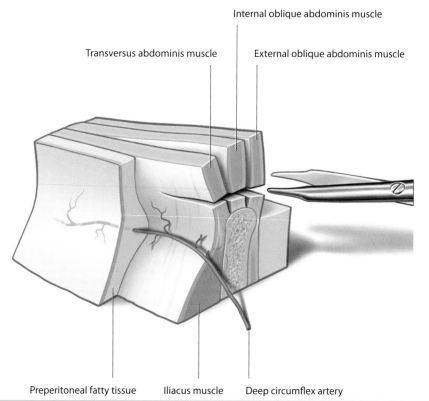

Internal oblique abdominis muscle

Transversus abdominis muscle

External oblique abdominis muscle

Preperitoneal fatty tissue

Iliacus muscle

Deep circumflex artery

Trimming of transversus and oblique muscles superior to DCIA

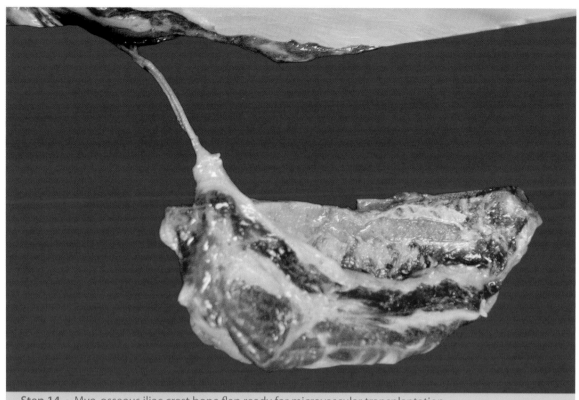

Step 14 • Myo-osseous iliac crest bone flap ready for microvascular transplantation

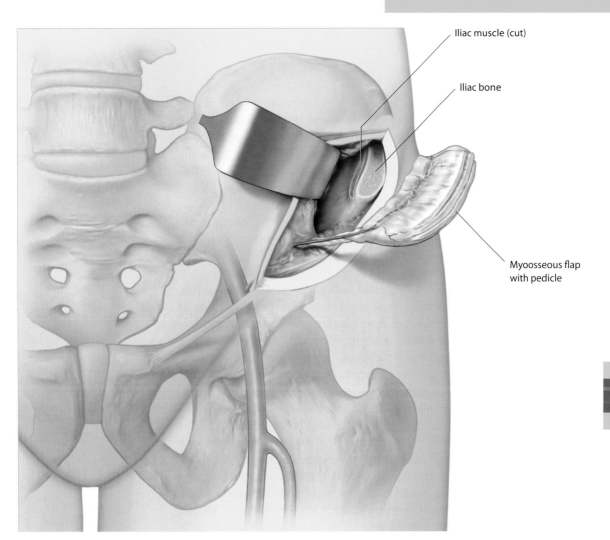

Iliac muscle (cut)

Iliac bone

Myoosseous flap
with pedicle

Flap perfusion is maintained until the recipient vessels are ready for anastomoses

Comments

Flap Design

For intraoral reconstruction, a skin paddle is only recommended in slim patients having significant and deep additional soft tissue defects, because the excess volume and bulk of the flap can lead to venous congestion of the skin paddle or functional discomfort for the patient. The skin paddle of the iliac crest osteocutaneous flap is more suitable for covering extra-oral or perforating defects.

Step 1: If the skin incision is made caudal to the line between the pubic tubercle and the ASIS, the femoral trigonum will be opened, and the dissection will be performed caudal to the vascular pedicle. Additionally, motor branches of the femoral nerve might be injured.

Step 3: After transection of the internal oblique muscle, the ascending branch of the DCIA might become visible first. This vessel should not be mistaken for the DCIA, but it will lead to the main artery if followed in a proximal direction. After having identified the DCIA, the ascending branch should still be left intact for anatomical orientation. Furthermore, this will give the chance to include parts of the internal oblique muscle for additional soft tissue cover.

Steps 5, 6: To facilitate osteotomy, wide exposure of the operating field is necessary. Therefore, the skin incision should be made at least 3 cm longer than the planned bone segment. If the hip is supported by a beanbag, access to the gluteal aspect of the pelvis is easier.

Step 7: Detachment of the gluteal muscles is best achieved using a sharp scalpel. The abdominal muscles can be bluntly undermined at the inner rim of the iliac crest, starting at the ASIS. Here, the DCIA can easily be followed as it courses along the undersurface of a muscle rim, which is formed by the iliacus and transversalis muscle.

Step 9: Before transection of the iliacus muscle and the inner periosteum of the pelvis, the pulse of the DCIA has to be palpated. Keeping a muscle cuff of about 1–1.5 cm is enough for reliable perfusion of the bone flap.

Steps 11, 12: Osteotomy should be completely performed using the oscillating saw instead of chisels. To obtain a parallel curved bone segment at both sides, the caudal osteotomy must follow the natural curve of the iliac crest. This can only be achieved if the soft tissues have been sufficiently detached from the gluteal aspect of the pelvis.

Step 13: Bone wax should be used to stop the diffuse bleeding from the cutting surface of the pelvis. No bone wax should be applied to the bone flap at the osteosynthesis margins.

Perforator Flaps

Development

With the increasing knowledge of vascular anatomy and the skin's blood supply and the refinement of surgical skills and instruments, the sophistication of free tissue transfer could develop further. The first precise descriptions of the structure of the integument and its vessels were given by Spateholz in 1893 [366], who even then made a distinction between direct and indirect cutaneous vessels (perforators) branching off from a source vessel. A detailed analysis of the fine blood vessels of the skin had already been published some years before by Manchot in 1889 [232]. He introduced vascular territories of the individual skin vessels, which later were further objectified by radiographic studies using lead oxide tincture injections [34]. On the basis of this knowledge, Esser was the first to build island flaps in which only the fine cutaneous perforators were preserved [34]. Although in times when cutaneous flaps were raised as random pattern flaps without knowledge of the specific anatomy of the skin, the vessel course at the skin was taken into consideration by McGregor, who described the first axial pattern skin flaps [34, 255]. Moreover, the significance of the muscles as carriers for cutaneous vessels was pointed out by Orticochea [34, 288], and the blood supply of the skeletal muscles of the human body was classified into five types by Mathes and Nahai [245]. They had already noted that in muscles with a dominant proximal pedicle (type I), a cutaneous side branch often could be found close to the muscle hilum. A further important contribution to the understanding of skin perfusion was made by Ponten [34]. In his paper, he emphasized the relevance of the deep fascia for skin perfusion and introduced the definition of fasciocutaneous flaps. A first classification of this type of flap was proposed by Cormack and Lamberty, who differentiated four types of fasciocutaneous flaps according to the number and course of the perforators, including osteomyofascial flaps (type D). An even more detailed definition of six different patterns of perforating vessels was provided by Nakajima, giving a description of the different vessel courses through muscle, septa, and subcutaneous fatty tissue [278]. Based on detailed anatomic dissections, dye injections and radiographic investigations, Taylor and Palmer introduced the angiosome concept, in which the blood supply of three-dimensional blocks of tissue is correlated with specific vessels. They described an angiosome as a composite block of tissue that is supplied anatomically by source vessels that span between the skin and bone. In addition to supplying the deep tissues, the source vessel of these angiosomes supplies branches to the overlying skin, which pass either between the deep tissues or through the deep tissues, usually muscle, to pierce the outer layer of the deep fascia. Hence, perforator flaps, when dissected to the underlying source vessels, involve tracing vessels either between the deep tissues, whether muscle, tendon, or bone, or through the deep tissues, usually muscle [380]. Thus, these three-dimensional tissue blocks can consist of all possible tissue components but are perfused by a single source vessel. Like vascular territories of the skin, adjacent angiosomes are connected by fine vascular anastomoses (choke anastomotic vessels).

The venous architecture was described as a continuous network of arcades that follow the body's connective tissue framework. It mirrors the arterial supply in the deep tissues, so that angiosomes consist of matching arteriosomes and venosomes [385].

A simplified classification of perforating vessels proposed by Hallock distinguishes direct from indirect perforators. Whereas the first travel directly from the source vessel through the subcutaneous fatty tissue to the skin and only penetrate the deep fascia, indirect perforators follow fascial spaces, intermuscular septa, or course through muscle tissue until they penetrate the deep fascia to reach the skin [281]. This simple classification finds general acceptance among surgeons [57]. Niranjan pointed out that indirect perforators can also travel through periosteum or tendons instead of muscle before they reach the skin, but this is only seldom the case [34].

Meanwhile, perforator flaps are harvested from many donor sites such as the anterolateral thigh [57, 194, 195, 215, 301], medial or lateral thigh [130, 207], the tensor fasciae latae [88, 193, 204], latissimus dorsi [186, 188, 211], rectus abdominis [8, 137, 205], and the gluteal region [6, 408], from the forearm [25, 325], the lower leg [56, 165, 201, 206, 208, 393], and many other regions of the body [103, 244].

Classification and Definition

Soft tissue flaps, perfused by defined singular vessels that penetrate the deep fascia, can be referred to as perforator flaps. They consist of skin and/or subcutaneous fatty tissue. The first description for a perforator flap without the source vessel was given by Koshima for the thinned paraumbilical perforator flap [205], and many others followed, describing numerous donor sites throughout the body. Following the simplified classification of Hallock, perforator flaps are named according to the course of the vessel penetrating the deep fascia. Thus, direct perforator flaps are perfused by a vessel running directly from the source artery to the deep fascia that they penetrate to enter the skin. Indirect perforator flaps are subdivided in myocutaneous or septocutaneous flaps, depending on the course of the vessel through muscle tissue or along intermuscular septa. Thus, to raise a perforator flap, the deep fascia must always be opened to follow the perforating vessel down to the source artery. Whereas in direct perforator flaps the dissection is performed only through fatty tissue, in indirect perforator flaps muscle fibers must be transected or separated (myocutaneous perforator flap), or at least one intermuscular septum must be opened (septocutaneous perforator flap). The individual perforator flap is then specified according to the name of the source vessel (deep inferior epigastric artery perforator flap) or according to the muscle that has to be separated (vastus lateralis perforator flap). Since the anastomosis of a perforator flap can either be performed without sacrifice of the source vessel at the perforating vessel itself (small-caliber short pedicle) or at the source vessel (large-caliber long pedicle), the structure of the vascular pedicle should be mentioned as a further characteristic of the flap (soleus perforator only flap, vastus lateralis long pedicle perforator flap). According to a definition by Kim, a perforator flap based on a musculocutaneous perforator should be named according to the name of the muscle perforated, and perforator flaps based on other types of perforators should be named according to the name of the proximal vessel. The term "perforator-based" should further define those flaps harvested without sacrificing the proximal vessels [187]. Therefore, the main difference with conventional flaps is that for elevation of a perforator flap, a specific skin vessel, the location of which can be variable, must be exposed and followed to the source vessel by incision of the deep fascia and, depending on its course, septa or muscle tissue. This technique allows for preservation of structures not needed for defect cover, particularly muscles including their motor innervation. Apart from the individual design of the skin flap, which can be exactly tailored to fit the defect, the major advantage of perforator flaps is their minimal donor site morbidity. However, for a successful reconstruction, mastering the subtle dissection required for flap raising, exact knowledge of the vascular anatomy and its possible variations, and reliable suturing of vessels with a diameter of 1 mm or less is mandatory.

Anterolateral Thigh Perforator Flap

159

Wolff/Hölzle, *Raising of Microvascular Flaps 2nd ed.*,
DOI: 10.1007/978-3-642-13831-7_8, © Springer-Verlag Berlin Heidelberg 2011

Development and Indications

When Song et al. published their paper in 1984 on the thigh as a donor site for three new flaps with the anterolateral thigh, they closely fulfilled all the characteristics of a perforator flap [361].

To raise the septocutaneous flap, opening the deep fascia and inclusion of the skin vessel located between the rectus and vastus lateralis muscle were specific components of the operating procedure. But other than elevating a true perforator flap according to the above-mentioned definitions, the conventional anterolateral thigh flap mostly includes a significant amount of subcutaneous fatty tissue. Often, a substantial portion of muscle tissue from the vastus lateralis is included in order to protect the perforating skin vessels and to guarantee a safe blood supply to the skin. Whereas initially the perforators were only visualized or partially exposed at the level of the deep fascia, they are now completely skeletonized along their course from the skin to the source vessel, which mostly is the descending branch of the lateral circumflex femoral artery. Doing this, any muscle tissue is discarded, and the subcutaneous fat is shaped or thinned according to the requirements of the defect. Moreover, different vascular pedicles arising from different source vessels can be used in the anterolateral thigh perforator flap, so that the flap can be raised in a freestyle approach as long as safe anastomosis is provided. After the first description by Song, it took several years until this flap became popular for different reconstructive purposes. With different focuses on the variety and shapes possible when using the conventional technique, a great number of clinical series with many different soft tissue reconstructions have been reported since the early 1990s. The flap has been used as a fasciocutaneous [117, 209, 354, 361, 419, 450], fascial [150], thinned skin flap [194, 195, 419, 429, 432], chimeric flap in combination with bone flaps [209, 419], muscle-only flap [423], myocutaneous flap [59, 89, 117, 191, 296, 419, 422, 423, 427] dermofat flap [59, 126, 161, 175, 433], and flow-through flap [12, 210] for reconstructions of the head and neck including the scalp, oral cavity, lips and esophagus, upper and lower extremities, foot and hand, trunk, female breast, abdominal wall, and other regions of the body. With this tremendous number of indications and clinical experience, the anterolateral thigh became a donor site for flaps that are primarily defined by the location, length, and course of its individual perforating vessel instead by the gross anatomical location of the skin island [235, 394].

Anatomy

Since the anatomy of the anterolateral thigh has already been described in Chap. 3, only a short review of the vascular anatomy with special regard to the perforating vessels is given here.

The superior part of the perforator flaps from the anterolateral thigh receive their blood supply from perforating vessels that arise from the descending branch of the circumflex femoral artery. Nevertheless, perforators can also arise from the transverse or the ascending branch of the lateral circumflex femoral artery or as a rare variation from an oblique branch or from the profunda or even the superficial femoral artery itself [12, 69, 190, 236, 354, 376, 436]. In 89 consecutive patients, Wong et al. found a mean 1.9 sizeable cutaneous perforators, which they identified as musculocutaneous perforators in 85% and septocutaneous vessels in 15% of all cases. Perforators located close to the septum have a short, direct intramuscular course [436]. The branching pattern of the skin vessels was described in a series of 74 clinical cases and could be classified into eight categories, but no variation was found making flap raising impossible. In this series, 2.3 perforators per case were found, 82% of them having a myocutaneous course, branching off at different levels from the descending branch [13, 190]. An oblique branch of the lateral circumflex femoral artery was noted to be present in 35% of cases, the source vessel for the dominant perforator in 14% of cases [436]. In addition to these variations of the source vessel, cutaneous branches may be absent in rare cases [69, 202, 215, 419, 422, 436], which was described to occur in up to 5.4% [190]. In the middle third of the thigh, the descending branch divides into a medial and a lateral branch in about 30% of patients. Whereas the medial branch gives off feeders to the rectus femoris muscle and the skin at the medial aspect of the thigh, the lateral branch is the source vessel for septo- or myocutaneous perforators to the skin of the anterolateral thigh. In a clinical study of 115 flap raising procedures at the anterolateral thigh, the descending branch was found to be absent in 22.6%, replaced by the medial descending branch or other strong muscle branches [13]. According to the results of anatomical investigations, the dominant cutaneous vessel of the anterolateral thigh was found to have a myocutaneous course in 60–80% [89, 190, 419, 422, 436], showing a septocutaneous pattern to be more frequent in the proximal part of the thigh [236]. In these cases, the dominant cutaneous vessel has a direct course to the skin, running along the intermuscular septum between the rectus femoris and vastus lateralis muscle and piercing the fascia lata without traversing through the vastus lateralis muscle. These flaps are raised without any muscle tissue and thus offer the possibility of raising thin and pliable skin paddles in slim patients, well suited for reconstructions in the head and neck area, including the oral cavity. The dominant cutaneous vessel can be found within a 4-cm radius at the midpoint of a line between the anterior superior iliac spine and the lateral border of the patella in nearly all patients [245, 424].

Apart from this main perforator, the descending branch gives rise to one to three additional cutaneous branches, reaching the skin more distally to the main perforator. Whereas the most distal vessels are not reliable for skin perfusion, a second perforator can be found in about 90% of all cases 4–9 cm distal to the main perforator, making it possible to build a second independent skin paddle. Like the dominant perforator, this additional cutaneous vessel has a myocutaneous course in 80–90% of individuals, piercing the muscle 2–5 cm from its medial rim [422, 424]; other authors describe a range of 0.1–7 cm, with a mean distance of 1.8 cm [230]. Because most of the perforators showing a myocutaneous course enter the muscle within 2–3 cm, only a small muscle cuff is necessary if the tedious dissection of these musculocutaneous perforators is not desired. Wong et al. investigated the course of the perforators in a series of 89 flaps and found perforators with a more lateral and distal location with a tortuous intramuscular course through the vastus lateralis [436]. A detailed description of the course of the perforators was given by Shieh et al., who classified them into four types according to their derivation and the direction in which they traversed the vastus lateralis muscle. In type I, vertical musculocutaneous perforators from the descending branch were found in 56.8% of patients, a mean 4.8 cm long. In type II, horizontal myocutaneous perforators from the transverse branch were found in 27%, 6.7 cm in length. Type III was found in 10.8% containing perforators with a vertical septocutaneous course from the descending branch with a mean length of 3.6 cm. In type IV (5.4%), horizontal septocutaneous perforators were found from the transverse branch, approximately 8 cm long [354].

Advantages and Disadvantages

Compared to the conventional anterolateral thigh flap (ALT) flap, which can include a significant amount of subcutaneous fatty tissue and muscle bulk, the meticulous dissection of the perforator allows the raising of thin and pliable flaps, individually designed according to the needs of the defect. Kimura and Satoh were the first to describe that vascular anatomy of the cutaneous perforators of the lateral thigh gives a suitable basis for primary flap thinning [194]. In their first five cases, they removed the subcutaneous fatty tissue uniformly from the whole flap except for the region around the perforator, obtaining a flap thickness of only 3–4 mm. Consequently, other authors also performed flap thinning if the perforator had a myocutaneous course. They used the perforator flap elevation technique and discarded the superfluous muscle tissue [49, 117, 419, 432]. Further experience has shown that the radical removal of fatty tissue does not impair flap perfusion, as long as the subdermal vascular plexus is preserved and attention is paid to the vascular territory of the corresponding flap vessels [203]. Although Ross and co-workers found a higher complication rate in their clinical series [315] and Alkureishi et al. could experimentally find a reduced dye perfusion of the thinned flaps [5], the literature generally reports low complication rates [5, 203, 419, 432, 442]. In an anatomic study by Nojima et al., the vascular territories of unthinned and thinned perforator flaps were compared by selectively injecting dye into the largest perforator of the descending branch. They found that the mean vascular territory of the unthinned flaps were 351 cm² and 256 cm² after thinning to a thickness to 6–8 mm. Hence, flap thinning led to a reduction to about 80% of the safe vascular territory [284]. In fresh cadavers, three- and four-dimensional computed tomographic angiography and venography showed changes in flap perfusion after thinning. The authors found that thinning reduces the size of the vascular territory by transecting recurrent vessels at the level of the suprafascial plexus [335]. Using three-dimensional imaging and latex dissections, these large-diameter linking vessels in the suprafascial level were also described by Saint-Cyr and co-workers. They pointed out that these vascular links enable perfusion of adjacent vascular territories and thus make it possible to raise extended flaps that are reliably perfused by a single dominant perforator [327]. All authors agree, however, that flap thinning must be performed by surgeons possessing high technical skills and exact knowledge of the vascular anatomy. If the subfascial vascular plexus is completely preserved, the size of the vascular territory of a thinned flap corresponds to conventional flaps [203, 275, 419].

One of the most important reasons for flap failure is the inadvertent division of the perforator at the fascial plane [57]. Thus, to reduce the uncertainty in predicting the anatomy of the perforators and to facilitate their exposure, preoperative mapping using an audible Doppler is generally recommended. Although the definite course of this dominant cutaneous vessel can only be explored during flap raising, a myocutaneous pattern can be expected if the Doppler signal is detected not directly between the rectus and vastus lateralis muscle, but 2–4 cm lateral to the septum. The use of the preoperative color Doppler assessment was investigated by comparing their intraoperative findings with the number and location marked by preoperative color Doppler flowmetry. Here, this method was found to have a high predictive value in prospective studies [170, 395]. On the other hand, sensitivity and specificity were found to be less reliable in audible Doppler and to be dependent on the type of hand-held Doppler used [184, 395, 448]. Rozen et al. proposed preoperative CT angiography, which provided better and more reliable information about the descending branch and its perforators compared to Doppler sonography. With this method, limbs with unsuitable perforators can be identified before surgery, and a better donor area can be selected [320].

The dissection of the perforators gives the opportunity to perform small-vessel anastomoses, if adequate small recipient vessels are present at the defect site. This can be helpful in patients with a paucity of conventional recipient vessels having had previous surgery. In these cases, only arteries with good pulsation may be selected, since otherwise no adequate flow will be established within the flap. If also an unconventional recipient vein is used it must be evident that this vein provides reliable drainage to the flap. It is mandatory that all such small vessels be handled with a high degree of sensitivity and great care to prevent vascular spasm and any kind of damage to the vessel wall. Because the sacrifice of the descending branch does not cause any disadvantage to the patient, it is generally recommended to raise a long pedicle ALT perforator flap and to make use of the long and high-caliber vascular pedicle it offers.

Flap Raising

Patient Positioning

Despite the anatomical variations described for the vascular pedicle of the anterolateral thigh/vastus lateralis flap, angiography is not helpful in locating the variable positions of the septo- or myocutaneous branches of the descending branch. Preoperative evaluation of the perforators should be performed using a Doppler probe by carefully auscultating the skin in the region of the intermuscular septum and over the medial parts of the vastus lateralis muscle. The patient is placed in a supine position, and the whole leg is included in the operating field to allow for free positioning of the extremity and for modifying the flap design, if necessary. Circular disinfection is performed from the hip down to the lower leg.

Flap Design

The skin paddle of the ALT perforator flap depends completely on the location of the perforator selected for flap raising. Thus, the definite design of the flap cannot be determined before a useful perforator shows that a strong pulsation has been exposed. This normally can be found a few centimeters proximal to the midpoint of the interconnection between the anterior superior iliac spine and the lateral rim of the patella. The longitudinal axis of the flap is designed parallel and 2–4 cm lateral to the septum between the rectus and vastus lateralis muscle. The length of the flap can reach up to 25 cm if the subfascial vascular network is preserved; flap width is limited to about 8 cm to allow for tension-free primary closure. When thinning the flap radically in the suprafascial plane, for safe perfusion it is recommended to keep the size of the flap within reasonable limits, not exceeding about 20×7 cm. The skin incision is marked medial to the tensor muscle at the proximal thigh and straight above the rectus muscle toward the knee, keeping a safe distance to the septum of about 3 cm.

The incision is made over the rectus femoris muscle, keeping a safe distance from the intermuscular septum, which can be palpated between the rectus and vastus lateralis muscles. The location of the septum is represented by the interconnecting line between the anterior superior iliac spine and the lateral border of the patella. The fascia lata still remains intact. Again it must be mentioned that before the skin paddle is outlined, the perforator(s) must be visualized in the subfascial plane to determine the center of the flap. The fascia is incised along the rectus femoris muscle and dissection is performed laterally to the intermuscular septum.

Step 1

Step 2

If no septocutaneous perforators are found, myocutaneous perforators will be present, which pierce the vastus muscle along its anterior border. This is the case in the majority of patients. Using magnifying glasses, these myocutaneous perforators become visible, entering the muscle along its undersurface at the anterior muscle rim. It can be helpful to retract the septum laterally using hooks.

Step 3

Because the perforators traverse the muscle closely underneath its surface, their pulsation can often be observed, and the tiny vessels can be followed easily from the skin paddle into the proximal direction by blunt separation of the muscle fibers.

Step 4

Under magnification, it can clearly be seen that the pedicle consists of one artery in the center and two comitant veins.

Step 5

The rectus femoris and vastus lateralis muscles are bluntly separated from each other, and by retracting the rectus femoris muscle medially, the descending branch of the circumflex femoral artery with its two comitant veins becomes visible. A vessel loop is placed around the artery and the comitant veins.

Step 6

The myocutaneous perforator is followed through the vastus lateralis muscle. Small side branches to the muscle are ligated or clipped, and the perforator is finally isolated with only a very small muscle cuff around it. Using magnifying glasses is strongly recommended to facilitate identification and dissection of the perforator.

Step 7

Definite determination of the flap margins is now possible since the perforator has been clearly visualized and dissected. The fascia is circumferentially incised while the perforator is safely protected.

Step 8

The skin paddle, which can now be designed in its final form, is raised completely.

Step 9

Flap raising is finished with further dissection of the perforator in the proximal direction, until the descending branch of the lateral circumflex femoral artery is reached. The descending branch is transected distal to the perforator, and the motor branch of the femoral nerve is left intact.

Step 10

The components of the perforator pedicle are separated from each other, and the flap is now ready for microvascular transplantation. Direct closure is possible if the width of the skin paddle does not exceed 8–9 cm. Burow triangles must be excised at the cranial and caudal flap pole to prevent formation of dog ears following linear closure.

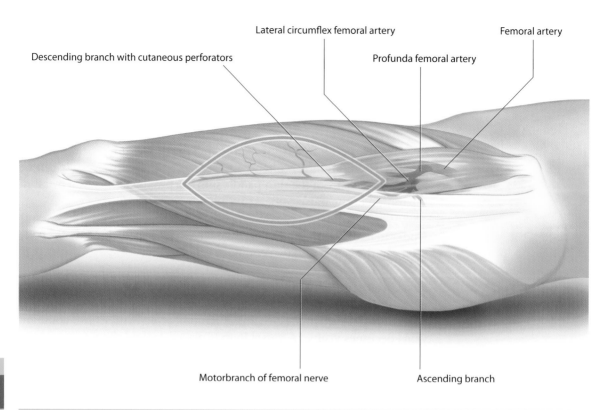

Lateral circumflex femoral artery

Femoral artery

Descending branch with cutaneous perforators

Profunda femoral artery

Motorbranch of femoral nerve

Ascending branch

Vascular system of the anterolateral thigh and standard skin paddle

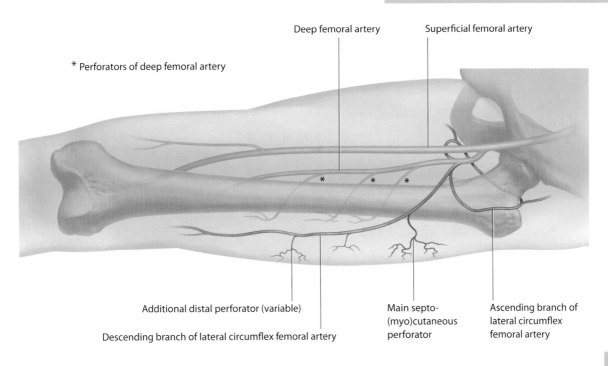

Deep femoral artery

Superficial femoral artery

* Perforators of deep femoral artery

Additional distal perforator (variable)

Descending branch of lateral circumflex femoral artery

Main septo-(myo)cutaneous perforator

Ascending branch of lateral circumflex femoral artery

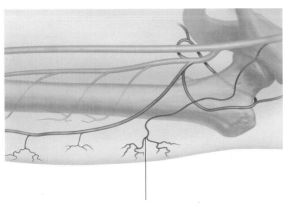

Variant of main septo-(myo)cutaneous perforator

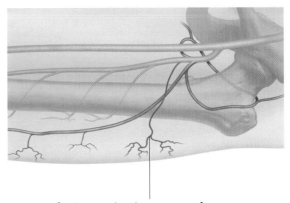

Variant of main septo-(myo)cutaneous perforator

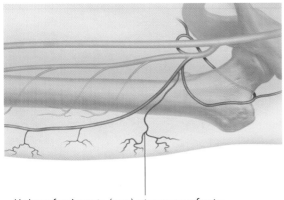

Variant of main septo-(myo)cutaneous perforator

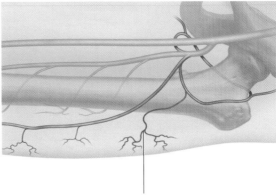

Variant of main septo-(myo)cutaneous perforator

Main septo- or myo-cutaneous perforator and variants

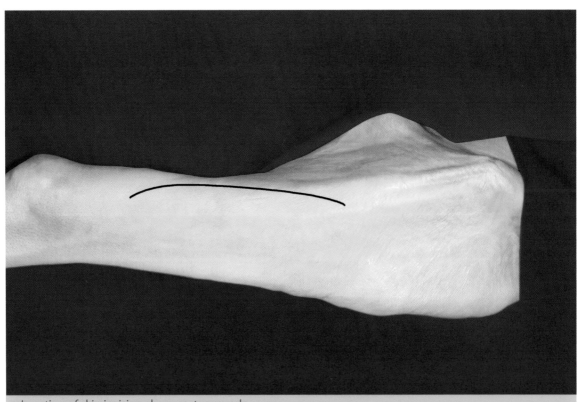

Location of skin incision above rectus muscle

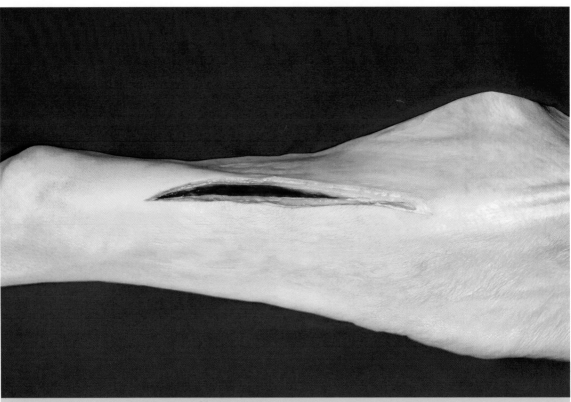

Step 1 • Skin incision and incision of fascia

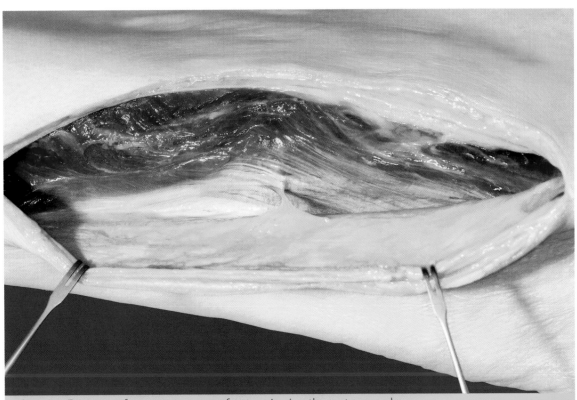

Step 2 • Exposure of myocutaneous perforator piercing the vastus muscle

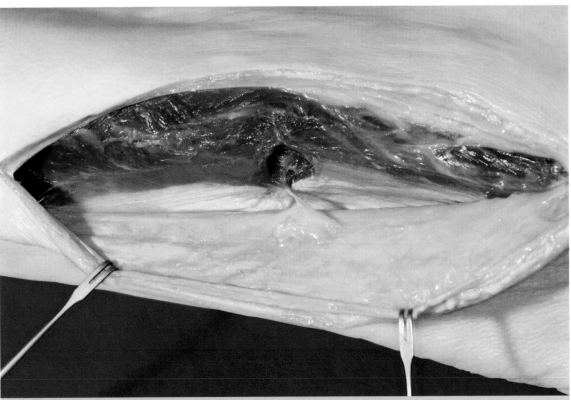

Step 3 • Blunt separation of muscle fibers

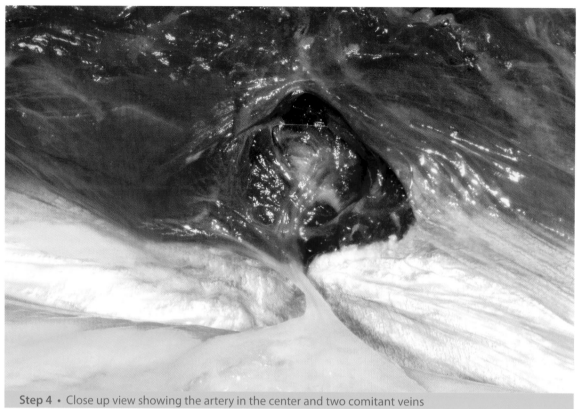

Step 4 • Close up view showing the artery in the center and two comitant veins

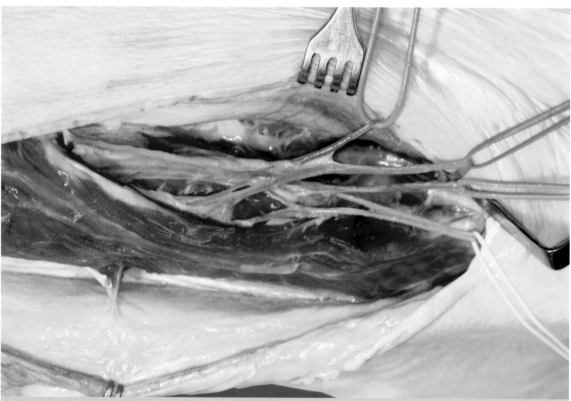

Step 5 • Exposure of the descending branch by retracting the rectus femoris muscle medially

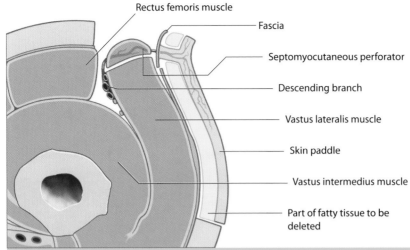

Rectus femoris muscle

Fascia

Septomyocutaneous perforator

Descending branch

Vastus lateralis muscle

Skin paddle

Vastus intermedius muscle

Part of fatty tissue to be deleted

Course of myocutaneous perforator, design of thinned flap

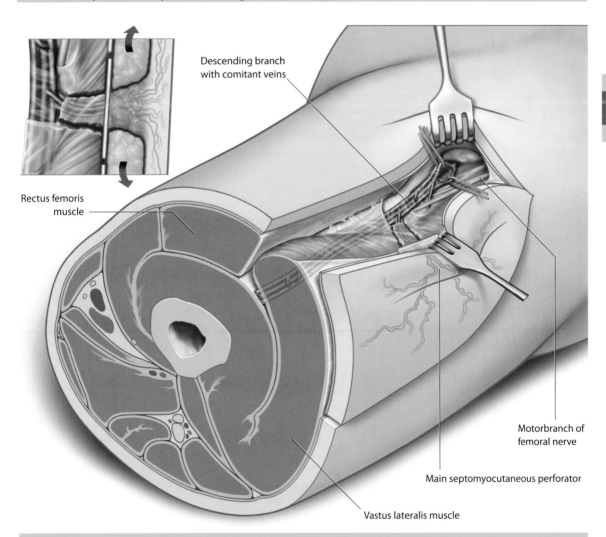

Descending branch with comitant veins

Rectus femoris muscle

Motorbranch of femoral nerve

Main septomyocutaneous perforator

Vastus lateralis muscle

Cross-section anatomy of the flap donor site
Inset shows cuff of muscle, fascia and fat around the perforator pedicle. Note the level of flap thinning.

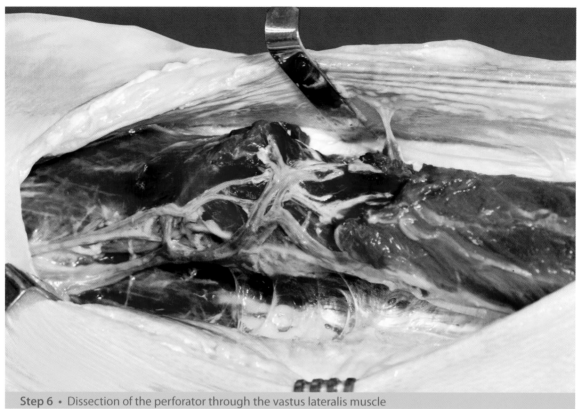

Step 6 • Dissection of the perforator through the vastus lateralis muscle

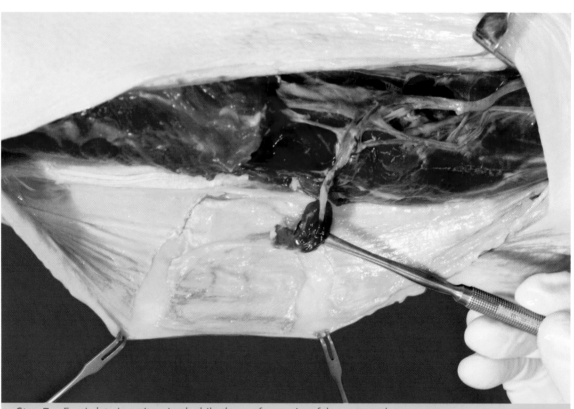

Step 7 • Fascia lata is peritomized while the perforator is safely protected

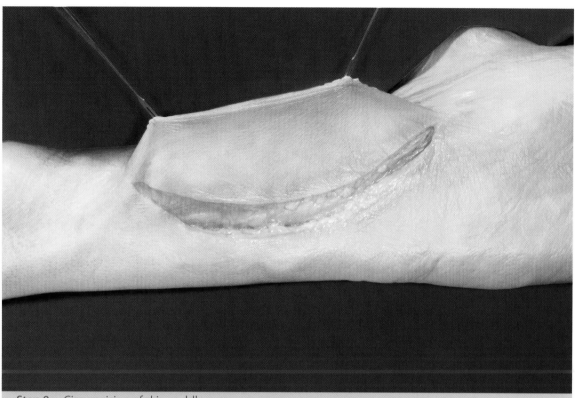

Step 8 • Circumcision of skin paddle

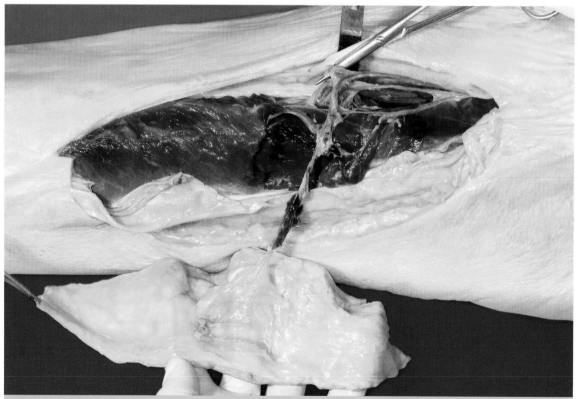

Step 9 • Further dissection of the perforator, transection of the descending branch

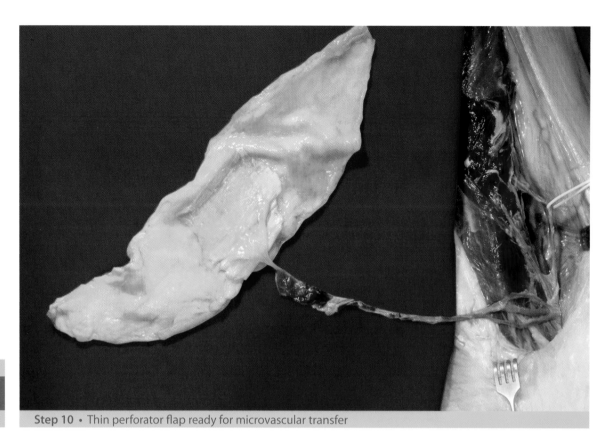

Step 10 • Thin perforator flap ready for microvascular transfer

Long pedicle perforator flap

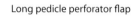

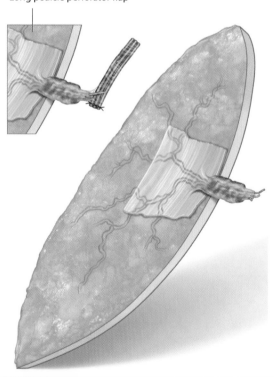

Short pedicle ("true") perforator flap. Patch of fascia protecting the vascular hilum

Comments

Planning

The skin island can never be outlined before the main perforating vessel is exposed. The skin incision to expose the main perforating vessel should not be outlined lateral to the rectus femoris muscle, because this will lead to injury of the intermuscular septum. Preoperative mapping of the main perforator using an audible Doppler can facilitate planning of the flap design.

Step 1: If the skin incision is performed too far laterally, the cutaneous perforator will be missed or injured. If the skin incision is performed too far medially, exposure of the descending branch may become difficult. For raising a perforator flap from the anterolateral thigh, it is easier when the perforator vessel branches off the descending branch, but it is not essential. We advise that the intermuscular septum be located preoperatively while the patient is extending the leg. If the fascia is incised medial to the rectus femoris muscle, the descending branch cannot be exposed. Palpate the rectus femoris muscle before the fascia is opened.

Steps 2–4: The perforator vessels, which run along the intermuscular septum, may easily be injured while opening the fascia. The use of magnifying glasses may facilitate identification and preservation of the perforators running along the septum. Detection of perforators can be alleviated when the septum is pulled laterally, and if the pulsation of the vessel is observed.

Step 6: The location, origin, and course of the perforators vary. In case of a myocutaneous course, perforator vessels may be injured if the muscle cuff around the perforator is too narrow. Keep a safe three-dimensional distance around these vessels while dissecting the muscular portion of the perforator.

Steps 7, 8: Before the skin paddle is outlined, locate the course of the perforator and the point where it perforates the fascia exactly.

Step 10: Blood flow can be different in the two veins accompanying the perforator artery. To determine the appropriate vein for anastomosis, venous return should be checked if possible before the pedicle is completely transected.

Soleus Perforator Flap

Wolff/Hölzle, *Raising of Microvascular Flaps 2nd ed.*,
DOI: 10.1007/978-3-642-13831-7_9, © Springer-Verlag Berlin Heidelberg 2011

The soleus perforator flap basically is a true perforator flap with a short pedicle, consisting of septo- or septomyocutaneous perforators on which anastomoses are performed. Thus, none of the main vessels of the lower leg has to be sacrificed. The perforators mostly arise from the peroneal vessels and are exposed at the proximal half of the lateral lower leg to allow for primary closure. Because of the similar anatomy of the skin paddle, the raising of this flap can easily be learned by surgeons familiar with the osteocutaneous fibular flap.

Before short pedicle perforator flaps such as the soleus perforator flap were established, free flaps from the lower leg were raised at the tibial posterior [449], tibial anterior [267, 415], and peroneal vessels [446], which served as the vascular pedicle. The tibial posterior flap was first described by Zhang et al. [449] as a distally based fasciocutaneous flap for defect cover at the foot and lower leg. In an anatomical study on 20 cadavers, the author found a high number of septocutaneous perforators coming from the tibial posterior artery. According to this study, three septocutaneous perforators from the posterior tibial artery can be found in the proximal, seven in the middle, and three in the distal lower leg. A precise description on the number and location of the septocutaneous branches of the tibial posterior artery was also given by Carriquiry and co-workers, who found four to five such perforators, each located 9–12, 17–19, and 22–24 cm above the medial ankle [54]. Amarante et al. used this flap as a distally pedicled transplant for defect cover at the foot, and they reported two regular branches that they found 4 and 6.5 cm above the medial ankle [9]. Similar findings were published by Koshima et al., who also preferred to raise flaps at the distal half of the lower leg due to the high number of septocutaneous perforators in this region [201]. To avoid sacrifice of this main vessel of the lower leg, they anastomosed their flaps directly to the perforator, leaving the tibial posterior artery intact [201]. Hung and co-workers later transferred this flap by means of microvascular anastomoses at the tibial posterior vessels for covering extended defects of the extremities [165]. A special indication of the free tibial posterior perforator flap was described by Chen et al., who performed reconstructions of the esophagus in three cases [60].

Focusing on the tibial anterior artery, based on their own cadaveric dissections Morrison and Shen described the proximal third of the lower leg to be the most reliable donor area for raising flaps based on septocutaneous perforators from this artery, each having a vascular territory covering 15×10 cm [267]. According to the first clinical applications, three types of tibial anterior flaps were described [267, 334, 415], all of them mainly used for local defect cover at the lower leg. The main advantages of flaps based on septocutaneous perforators from the tibial anterior artery are their wide arch of rotation, their thinness, and the ease of flap raising, making them an ideal transplant for defect cover at the foot [267].

Although Yoshimura et al. described the possibility of raising cutaneous flaps on the peroneal vessels early [445–447], only a few publications have reported on the usefulness of this flap until now. This paucity of clinical applications can be explained by the fact that cutaneous perfusion by the perforating vessels was reported to be unreliable [51, 54, 406], the localization of perforators to be extremely variable [51, 343], and the exposure of the peroneal vessels with an intact fibula to be difficult [286, 406]. The demanding technique in raising the peroneal flap and the general disadvantage of sacrificing one of the main arteries when using conventional flaps in the lower leg led to further modifications in flap design. With the development of perforator flaps on other regions of the body, the lower leg was also taken into consideration as a donor site for perforator flaps with a short pedicle. Since the anatomy of the cutaneous perforators was well known from the above-mentioned studies, it was only a small step to raise short-pedicle true perforator flaps without sacrificing the source vessels. The small cutaneous vessels in these types of flaps are traced to the source artery by retrograde dissection, so that adequate pedicle length and diameter for anastomosis can be obtained [430, 434].

Anatomy

179

Numerous anatomical studies have been conducted to investigate the number and course of the cutaneous branches of the peroneal artery. In dissections on 80 cadavers, Schusterman and co-workers [343] found 3.74 cutaneous perforators from the peroneal artery, 1.3 of them showing a septocutaneous, and 1.9 a myocutaneous vessel course; a mean 0.6 vessels were adherent at the fascia between the soleus and the peroneus muscles without piercing these muscles. For the osteocutaneous fibula flap, Schusterman proposed including the whole septum because of the variability of perforators. Yoshimura, who first described the peroneus flap, found 4.8 cutaneous branches, 71% of them having a myocutaneous course through the flexor hallucis and soleus muscles [445]. Whereas Yoshimura proposed raising the skin paddle more distally, other authors consider the middle third of the lower leg to be the safest donor area for the skin flap. Further anatomical studies in 30 cadavers showed that a mean 4.2 perforating vessels branch off from the peroneal artery to the skin, tending to run myocutaneously in the proximal third and septocutaneously in the distal third of the lower leg [430]. As with the main arteries, perforators at the lower leg consist of one artery and two concomitant veins and pierce the strong crural fascia. Although the localization of the cutaneous branches is generally quite variable, Wolff et al. found that the most proximally and distally located perforating vessels are the most uniform. These are consistently found in an area 5–15 cm below the fibula head and in the distal third of the lower leg 8–12 cm above the lateral ankle. To make direct closure of the donor site possible, the donor area in the proximal half of the lower leg is preferred; here, the perforators have a course through the soleus muscle. Selective dye injections have shown that one perforating vessel supplies an average cutaneous area of 12×7 cm, which is large enough for a number of reconstructive purposes [430]. To identify the course of the vessels, the perforators must be traced to their origin from the main arteries. In their anatomical study as well as in their clinical cases, the perforators originated exclusively from the peroneal artery, most of them having a course through the flexor hallucis and soleus muscles; in only 18%, the perforators coursed directly to the skin. Due to the deep location of the peroneal artery and the broad posterior intermuscular septum, the length of the perforators was at least 4–5 cm, and the diameter of the vessels varied between 1 and 1.5 mm for the arteries and 1.5 and 2.5 mm for the veins. Additional small branches from the perforator to the surrounding muscles enable the dissection of a well-perfused muscle cuff; no direct branch to the periosteum or fibula bone was found to originate from the perforators.

Based on a dissection of 20 cadaver legs, Heitmann et al. described 4.8 perforators of the peroneal artery with an external diameter at the posterior border of the fibula between 0.3 and 1.5 mm, for a mean 0.6 mm [148]. In an early report, Weber and Pederson showed the feasibility of connecting such small vessels when they salvaged the skin paddle of the osteoseptocutaneous fibular flap by performing independent microvascular anastomoses at the perforators in two osteocutaneous fibular flaps [414]. A similar report was published by Yokoo and co-workers who pointed out that this type of maneuver can also become necessary in osteomyocutaneous fibular flaps, if the perforator of the skin paddle as a variation branches off from the tibialis posterior instead of from the peroneal vessels [444]. As a consequence of these clinical experiences, Wong et al. conducted an anatomical study to evaluate the use of the soleus musculocutaneous perforator for skin paddle salvage in such situations. In 18 of 20 limbs, they found one or more musculocutaneous perforators at least 0.5 mm in diameter, located within 6 cm of the junction between the middle and lower third of the fibula. In this study, only 50% of the perforators originated from the peroneal artery, and in 35% from the tibial posterior vessels so that the authors suggested preserving one or two soleus perforators during harvest of the osteocutaneous fibular flap until existence of the septocutaneous perforator is confirmed [435]. A three-dimensional analysis in eight cadavers using an injection of a mixture of lead oxide and gelatin revealed a mean 13 perforators, originating from the peroneal, popliteal, and tibial posterior vessels; each perforator supplied an area of about 38 cm^2 [375]. Clinical applications of perforator flaps from the lateral lower leg were also described by Kawumara and co-workers. They published their experience with free soleus and free peroneal perforator flaps in 23 patients without sacrificing any of the main arteries in the lower leg. The perforator pedicle length varied between 6 and 10 cm in soleus perforator flaps, with the largest skin paddle being 15×9 cm, and 4 and 6 cm in peroneal perforator flaps. The maximum size of the skin paddle was 9×4 cm; only one flap was lost in this series [182].

Advantages and Disadvantages

Previous anatomical studies have shown that the skin of the lower leg is supplied by perforators from all three main vessels [54, 267, 375, 415], and this led to the development of free skin flaps from the tibial anterior [267, 332], tibial posterior [9, 182, 201], and peroneal system [430, 447]. To avoid sacrificing the main artery, tibialis posterior and medial sural [182] free perforator flaps were raised and anastomosed directly on the perforating vessel. These true perforator flaps were mainly used for defect cover in the extremities. In a publication by Tsai and co-workers, a free lateral leg perforator flap was used for reconstruction in a patient with an extended anterior cervical scar contracture [393]. In this case, a 22×8-cm² skin flap was elevated from the whole lateral aspect of the lower leg and was based on two myocutaneous perforators that joined approximately 2 cm below the fibula head. Because the vascular anatomy of the lateral lower leg has meticulously been investigated in previous studies [54, 343, 375, 445] and is also well known from the osteomyocutaneous fibula transfer, exposure of the perforators and flap raising is possible without technical difficulties. Although strong perforators can also be found in the distal third of the lower leg [9, 444], choosing a more proximal donor site is recommended because here direct wound closure is possible for a flap width of up to about 7 cm. Other than with the fibula or peroneus flaps, in which the peroneal artery is sacrificed, no preoperative diagnostics is necessary in the soleus perforator flap to exclude anatomical variations in the course of the major arteries of the lower leg. Therefore, in the conventional flaps of the lower leg, an important part of surgical planning is angiography, which allows visualization of variations and arteriosclerotic damage of the major vessels. In the soleus perforator flap, the only preoperative measure that can facilitate flap raising is the use of an audible or color-coded Doppler, which can help locate the perforator exactly. Especially when small flaps are planned, preoperative mapping of the perforators with the Doppler or the more precise color Doppler duplex imaging [134, 303] is helpful to place the first incision at a distance of approximately 2–3 cm from the vessel, so that after flap raising has been completed, it will be located in the center of the skin paddle. Of great importance for successful flap transfer is performing anastomosis without tension on the pedicle. Therefore, this type of flap is only recommended if recipient vessels can be expected close to the defect region. In patients with a deficiency of neck vessels, the reverse flow facial artery was proposed as a recipient vessel for such short pedicle perforator flaps [159]. Apart from the minimal donor site morbidity, the soleus perforator flap is primarily thin and pliable because it only carries a thin layer of subcutaneous fatty tissue. Thus, it is considered to be more suitable for intraoral reconstruction [430, 434] than perforator flaps from other donor sites that might need additional thinning.

The main disadvantage of short pedicle perforator flaps is that they have to be anastomosed at their short and small-diameter vessels, and anastomosing these vessels requires special technical skill [203, 417]. Thus, mastering small 1-mm vessel anastomoses is a prerequisite for any surgeon intending to do a short pedicle perforator flaps. Moreover, subtle dissection of the small vessels is mandatory to prevent vascular spasm. It is therefore strongly recommended to choose tall and slim patients for the first perforator flaps, because here greater vessels can be expected, which will facilitate dissecting and anastomosing the pedicle.

Flap Raising

Patient Positioning

The leg is bent into the knee joint at a right angle and brought in a lateral decubitus position for better access to the lateral and posterior aspect of the calf. This is facilitated by supporting the hip with a beanbag. The entire lower extremity is prepped circumferentially, and the foot is draped leaving the foot pulses accessible. A tourniquet should not be used, because it would make identification of the strength and pulse of the perforator impossible. Preoperative auscultation of the region of the posterior intermuscular septum with a Doppler probe will help locate the most suitable perforator.

Flap Design

The location of the skin paddle of the soleus perforator flap is completely dependent on the perforator selected for flap raising. Therefore, the design of the flap cannot be determined before a useful perforator showing a strong pulsation has been exposed. The perforator normally can be found a few centimeters distally to the fibular head and 1–3 cm posterior to the septum between the peroneal and soleus muscle. The longitudinal axis of the flap is designed parallel to the septum; the length of the flap can reach up to 15 cm if a strong and pulsatile perforator has been found; flap width is limited to about 6–7 cm which is the limit for tension-free primary closure. The skin incision is marked above the peroneal muscle, keeping a safe distance to the septum of about 2 cm. To prevent injury to the common peroneal nerve, a distance of about 4 cm is maintained to the fibular head.

Depending on the location of the perforator found by preoperative mapping, the incision is slightly curved anteriorly. A longitudinal skin incision is made proximal at the lower leg, beginning 4–5 cm distal to the fibula head along the peroneus longus muscle. A distance of 2 cm to the posterior intermuscular septum is kept, which can easily be palpated posterior to the muscle.

Step 1

The strong crural fascia is incised, and the perforator is visualized by carefully separating the fascia from the peroneal muscles and by blunt dissection in the posterior direction.

Step 2

Step 3

The posterior intermuscular septum, which covers the perforator from both sides, is exposed and then incised sharply along the lateral margin of the fibula without harming the perforator.

Step 4

To obtain better access to the deep flexor space, the peroneal muscles are retracted anteriorly and the soleus muscle is retracted posteriorly using hooks after detaching the muscle from the fibula. Dorsal to the fibula bone, the flexor hallucis longus muscle becomes visible, and the common peroneal nerve is looped.

Step 5

If two or more perforators can be found, the strongest is selected to perfuse the flap. Using magnifying glasses, the perforator artery together with the two comitant veins are then traced directly to the peroneal vessels. In the perfused leg, the artery can easily be palpated at the posterior aspect of the fibula. If the perforator pierces the soleus or the flexor hallucis longus muscle, which is the case in the majority of patients, an intramuscular dissection is performed, and the few tiny muscular branches are carefully clipped.

Step 6

The peroneal vessels can be carefully exposed and looped distal to the perforator. This facilitates access to the perforator origin from the source vessels.

Step 7

The skin paddle is now circumcised to the level of the crural fascia, which is included to protect the perforating vessel. The skin paddle is raised such that the perforating vessel is located in the center of the flap. The size of the flaps can reach up to 6×12 cm.

Step 8

Flap raising is completed. Perforator vessels are clipped at their origin from the peroneal vessels, which are left intact. After drain insertion, wound closure is easily achieved by blunt mobilization of the edges. If needed, the Burow triangles are excised to prevent dog-ear formation, so that a straight scar without any contour irregularities is obtained. Postoperative immobilization of the patient is not necessary.

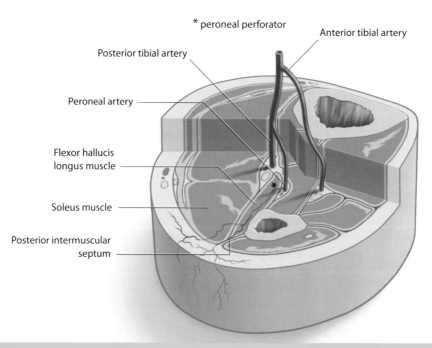

* peroneal perforator

Anterior tibial artery

Posterior tibial artery

Peroneal artery

Flexor hallucis longus muscle

Soleus muscle

Posterior intermuscular septum

Cross-section anatomy showing the course of the peroneal perforator along flexor hallucis muscle and posterior intermuscular septum. An additional branch is sent to the soleus muscle

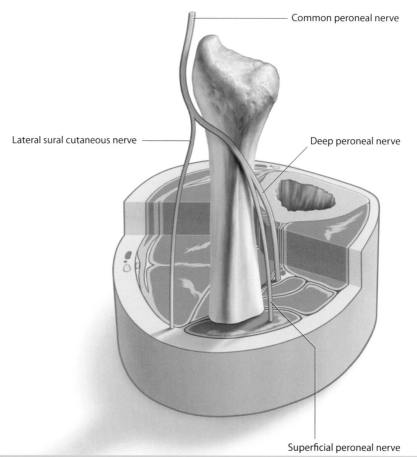

Common peroneal nerve

Lateral sural cutaneous nerve

Deep peroneal nerve

Superficial peroneal nerve

Cross-section anatomy of branches of the common peroneal nerve

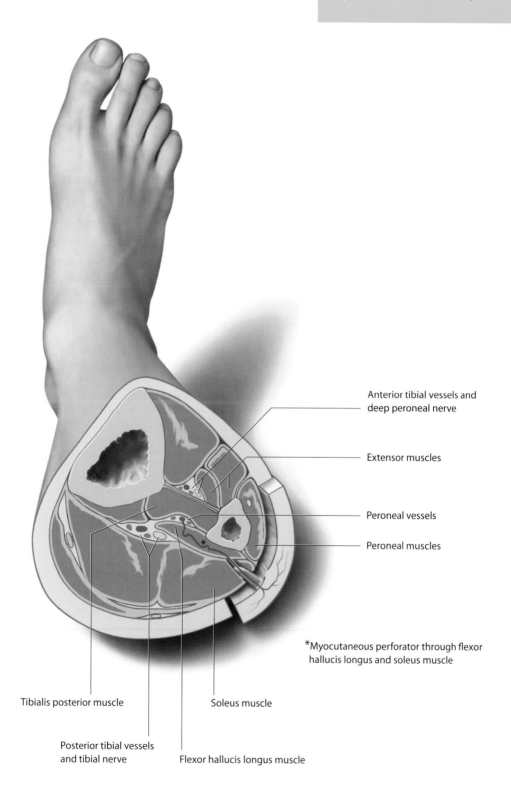

Anterior tibial vessels and deep peroneal nerve

Extensor muscles

Peroneal vessels

Peroneal muscles

*Myocutaneous perforator through flexor hallucis longus and soleus muscle

Tibialis posterior muscle

Soleus muscle

Posterior tibial vessels and tibial nerve

Flexor hallucis longus muscle

Cross-section anatomy of the soleus perforator flap and donor site

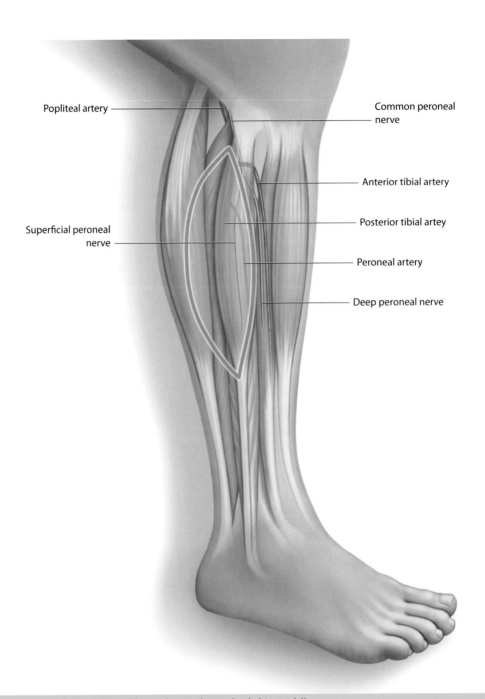

Popliteal artery

Common peroneal nerve

Anterior tibial artery

Posterior tibial artey

Superficial peroneal nerve

Peroneal artery

Deep peroneal nerve

Vascular system of the proximal lower leg and standard skin paddle

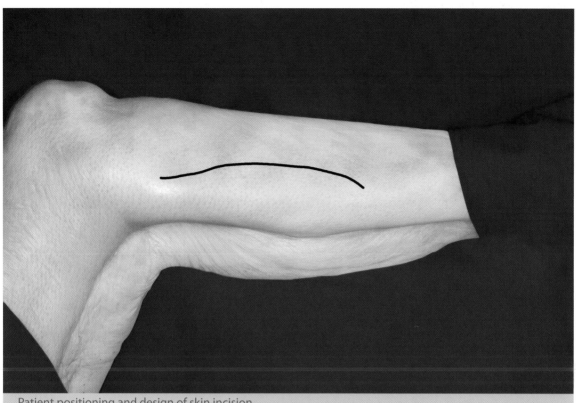

Patient positioning and design of skin incision

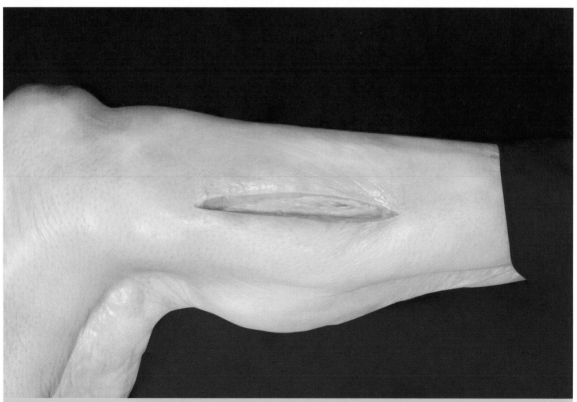

Step 1 • Incision of skin as far as crural fascia

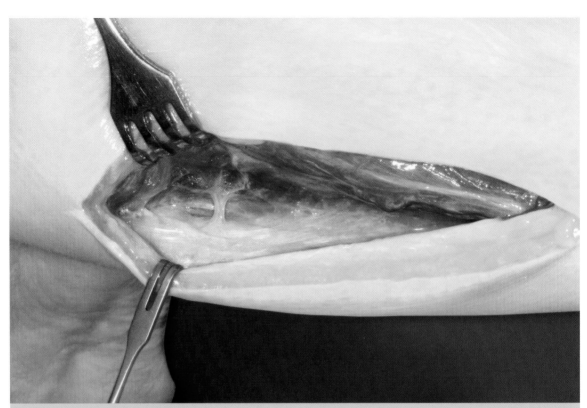

Step 2 • The perforator is visualized by carefully separating the fascia from the peroneal muscles and blunt dissection in posterior direction

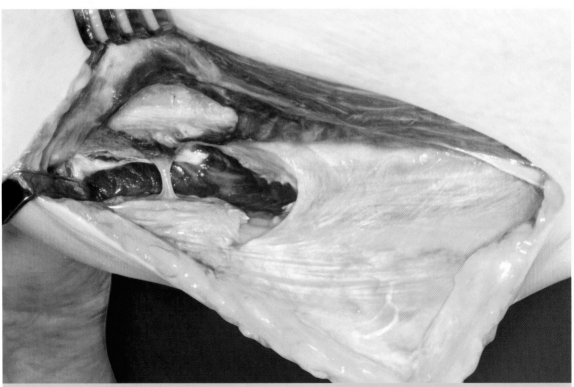

Step 3 • Incision of the posterior intermuscular septum

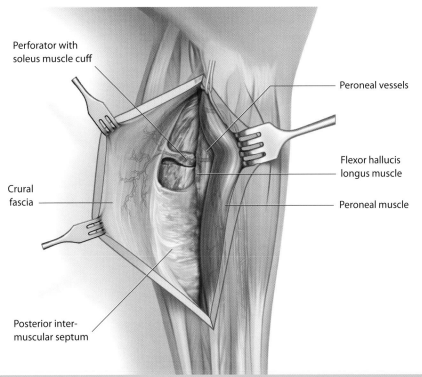

Perforator with
soleus muscle cuff

Peroneal vessels

Crural
fascia

Flexor hallucis
longus muscle

Peroneal muscle

Posterior inter-
muscular septum

Exposure of the perforator with muscle cuff. The posterior intermuscular septum is transected parallel to the pedicle, and the crural fascia is maintained at the undersurface of the skin

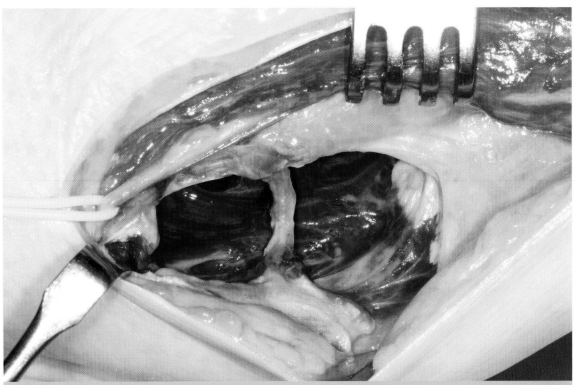

Step 4 • For better access to the deep flexor space, the peroneal muscles are retracted anteriorly and the soleus muscle is retracted posteriorly

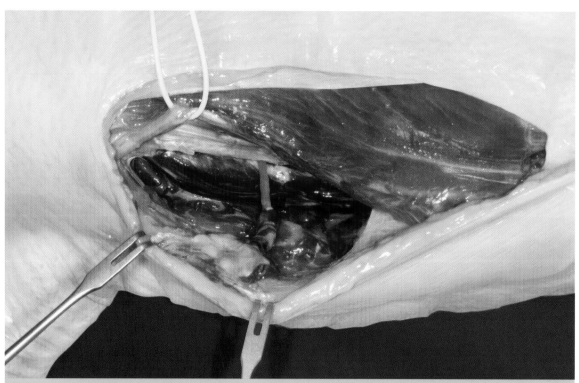

Step 5 • Perforator is dissected up to the peroneal vessels, leaving a small cuff of muscle around the perforator before it pierces the fascia

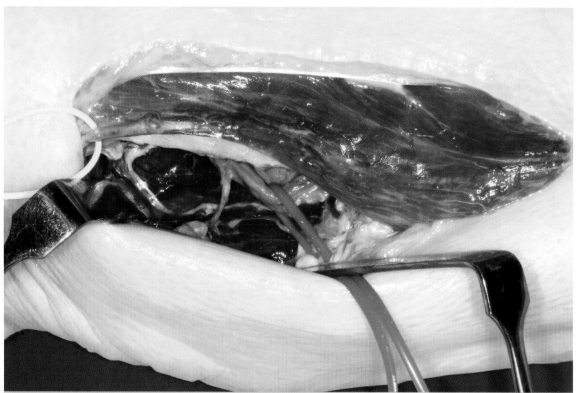

Step 6 • Dissection of perforator artery and veins directly to the peroneal vessels (looped)

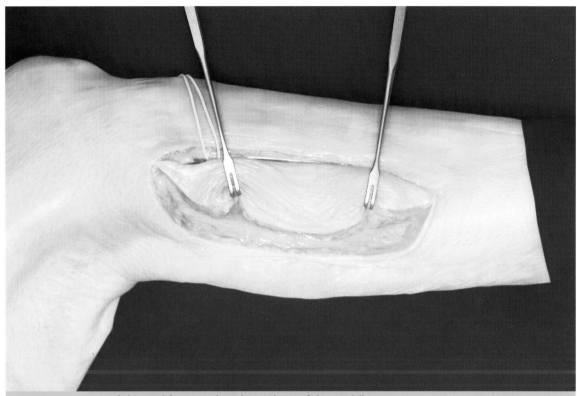

Step 7 • Incision of skin and fascia at dorsal periphery of skin paddle

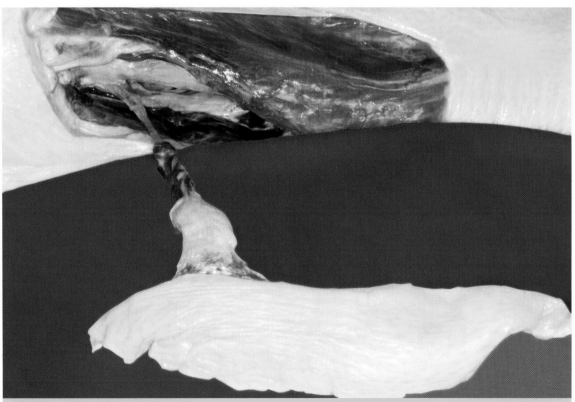

Step 8 • Flap raising is completed

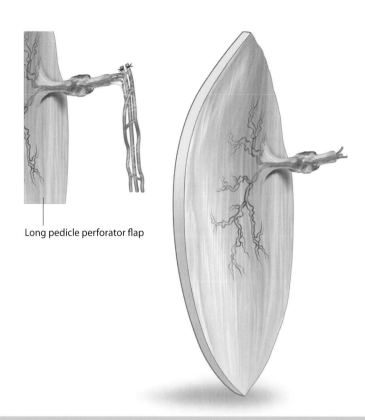

Long pedicle perforator flap

Schematic drawing of the vascular anatomy. With inclusion of the source vessels, a long pedicle peroneal perforator flap can be obtained

Comments

Flap Design

The posterior intermuscular septum is the key structure to design the skin paddle. Sometimes it is mistaken with the anterior intermuscular septum, which is located between the peroneus and the extensor muscles. The posterior intermuscular septum can easily be identified by palpating the groove between the Achilles tendon and peroneus muscles above the ankle, which can then be followed proximally.

Step 1: The skin island can never be outlined before the main perforating vessel is exposed. The skin incision should not be made over or lateral to the posterior intermuscular septum, because in this case, the perforator will be missed. Preoperative mapping of the main perforator using an audible Doppler can facilitate planning the flap design.

Step 2: The posterior intermuscular septum should be opened carefully to expose the perforator.

Step 4: Especially in the common case of a myocutaneous perforator, these vessels must be carefully dissected on their course through the soleus and flexor hallucis muscles. Note that the cutaneous perforator regularly sends a branch to the peroneal muscles so that bleeding will occur when forming a small muscle cuff. Keep a distance of about 1 cm from the cutaneous branch to be able to cauterize the muscle bleeding without damaging the skin vessel.

Step 7: The sural nerve and posterior saphenous vein may become exposed at the distolateral periphery of the skin flap and might be ligated, if necessary.

Step 8: To facilitate elevation of the flap, hold the skin paddle between two fingers to protect the perforator from both sides. In case of a myocutaneous perforator, leave a small cuff of soleus muscle along the vessel, with its greatest thickness of about 1 cm around the perforator.

Deep Inferior Epigastric Artery Perforator Flap

Wolff/Hölzle, *Raising of Microvascular Flaps 2nd ed.*,
DOI: 10.1007/978-3-642-13831-7_10, © Springer-Verlag Berlin Heidelberg 2011

Development and Indications

The first report of flap raising procedures at the anterior abdominal wall including parts of the rectus muscle was given by Brown et al., who described the myocutaneous rectus abdominis flap as a pedicled flap [47]. This report was followed by the first microvascular transfer with anastomoses to the deep inferior epigastric vessels performed by Pennington and Pelly [292]. Before this, the significance of the perforating vessels of the rectus muscle was emphasized by Holstrom (1979) and Robbins (1979). The superficial epigastric vascular system was already used as a source for free skin flaps raised from the lower abdomen and groin region by Antia and Buch (1971) [11] and Taylor and Daniel (1975) [381]. Both the deep and the superficial systems have partially overlapping vascular territories and are connected by choke arteries. Of these, the paraumbilical perforators originating from the deep system are the strongest and therefore contribute most to skin perfusion of the anterior abdominal wall [33, 46, 116]. Very soon after the first descriptions, a number of different flap designs and orientations of the skin paddle were described, all confirming the unique usefulness of myocutaneous flaps from the deep inferior vascular system. The main indication for this conventional myocutaneous flap, which includes significant parts of the rectus abdominis muscle, is breast reconstruction, but it is also used for other regions of the body such as the skull base, face, head and neck, trunk, and extremities [48, 95, 97, 143, 264, 384, 402, 404, 438]. It soon became clear that the sacrifice of parts of the rectus muscle, especially with removal of the anterior rectus sheath, can lead to complications such as weakness of the abdominal wall with herniation or bulging; therefore, several techniques were described for closure of the muscle defect by direct approximation [143, 402] using turnover flaps from the contralateral rectus sheath [259] or inserting synthetic material into the muscle defect created [95, 221].

With the introduction of the inferior epigastric artery perforator flap without the rectus abdominis muscle, this disadvantage was overcome. After identifying a strong perforating vessel, Koshima left all the rectus muscle tissue intact when he followed the perforator to the deep epigastric system by gently spreading the muscle fibers. This procedure first met all the criteria of raising perforator flaps according to the current definition [200]. The attractiveness of this procedure was further increased when the same author introduced the technique of primary flap thinning, which became possible with the targeted dissection and preservation of the perforator, allowing for safe removal of all superfluous fatty tissue [205]. As with the conventional transverse rectus abdominis (TRAM) or rectus abdominis flaps, these deep inferior epigastric perforator flaps were still anastomosed to the deep inferior epigastric vessels [7, 116]. If there is a need to extend the flap to the contralateral side of the abdomen, which is regularly the case in breast reconstruction, a perforator from the contralateral side can additionally be anastomosed to the end of the ipsilateral deep inferior epigastric vessels, thus increasing the safety of the blood supply (supercharging technique) [116, 293]. This technique is also useful in the presence of vertical scars, which can reduce blood circulation contralateral to the side of the anastomoses [341]. A similar technique was also described by Blondeel and Boeckx who additionally used contralateral perforators, which they anastomosed to the internal thoracic vessels instead of using the ipsilateral main vessels of the flap alone [32].

The first anastomoses of a deep inferior epigastric perforator flap exclusively to its perforating vessels was again performed by Koshima et al., describing this technique as supramicrosurgery [203]. Moreover, they recognized another significant advantage of perforator flaps, namely the possibility of primary radical flap thinning. Indications of those superthin perforator flaps with a short pedicle were superficial skin defects of the lower extremities, scalp, abdomen, or head and neck [203, 347, 374, 443].

Anatomy

Together with the oblique muscles, the rectus abdominis muscle forms the anterior abdominal wall; when raising a DIEAP flap, this muscle is nearly completely left unaffected. The rectus muscle, which originates from the cartilaginous parts of the sixth, seventh, and eighth ribs and the xiphoid process, is subdivided into four components by tendinous inscriptions. At its insertion at the pubic bone, it is covered by the pyramidalis muscle in about 80% of individuals. The muscle is enveloped into the rectus sheath, which forms the muscle-free linea alba at the midline. This muscle fascia is anteriorly built by the tendinous fibers of the external oblique and the anterior parts of the internal oblique abdominis muscle. Posteriorly, the internal oblique together with the transversalis muscle forms the posterior rectus sheath cranial to the arcuate line. The arcuate line is located on each side with a cranial convex orientation between both anterior superior iliac spines and the midline. Caudal to this line, there is no posterior component of the rectus sheath. Also on both sides, the linea semilunaris marks the lateral border of the rectus muscle, reaching from the lower ribs to the pelvis. Here, the segmental nerves coming from the terminal branches of the lower six intercostal nerves penetrate the posterior rectus sheath about 3 cm medial to the linea semilunaris. They provide motor innervation to the rectus muscle as well as sensory innervation to the abdominal skin. These mixed nerves run between the transverse and internal oblique muscles.

The blood supply to the abdominal skin and the rectus muscle, which according to the classification of Mathes and Nahai has a type III perfusion, derives from the deep inferior epigastric artery (DIEA) and two comitant veins, running at the posterior surface of the muscle within the rectus sheath. Cranial to the umbilicus, the vessels anastomose with the deep superior epigastric vessels, which develop from the internal thoracic vessels; thus, the deep superior epigastric artery (DSEA) can also be used as the source vessel [136, 282]. The DIEA branches off from the external iliac artery opposite the deep circumflex iliac artery (DCIA). It runs extraperitoneally in a medial and cranial direction, and after reaching the lateral rim of the rectus muscle, the pedicle penetrates the transversalis fascia about 3–4 cm caudal to the arcuate line [399]. The vessels enter the rectus muscle at its undersurface mostly at its middle (78%), seldom at its distal (17%) or proximal (5%) third [262]. With a diameter of 2–4.5 mm, both artery and veins have a large caliber, and the extramuscular length of the pedicle is a mean 10 cm [34]. In most cases, the veins unify before joining the external iliac vein. Boyd and co-workers have shown that the DIEA dominantly provides blood flow to the anterior abdominal wall. Apart from the continuation to the deep superior epigastric artery (DSEA), the vessel anastomoses cranially with branches of the intercostal arteries, and laterally and caudally, anastomoses exist with the superficial inferior epigastric artery (SIEA) and the DCIA via multiple choke arteries. The branches of the periumbilical perforators radiate in any direction of the abdominal skin, thus making it possible to harvest flaps with virtually any orientation [399]. However, according to the anatomical work by Taylor, the dominant orientation of the subdermal vascular network is 45° from the horizontal [381, 399], which makes an oblique design of the skin paddle most reliable.

Based on the clinical experience in his first 16 unipedicled TRAM flaps, Hartrampf described four perfusion zones for the lower abdomen, which have been adopted for the free TRAM as well as for the free DIEAP flap. When using a transverse skin paddle extending to both sides of the abdomen, four flap zones are defined: zone I lies ipsilateral over the rectus muscle and zone III ipsilateral and lateral to the linea semilunaris; according to this, the location of zones II and IV are contralateral to the side of the pedicle. Contrast injection studies have confirmed the clinical experience that the blood supply of zone IV is the most tenuous [181]. Using laser-induced fluorescence of indocyanine green, Holm et al. found decreased or no perfusion in zone IV and best perfusion in zones I and III [157]. Moreover, selective dye injections have shown that zones I–III are regularly supplied by a single perforating vessel, whereas zone IV was only partially or not stained [149]. The anatomy and blood flow of the DIEA were investigated in detail by Blondeel and co-workers [32, 33, 116]. They showed that in about 75% of subjects, the DIEA divides into two branches, the lateral of which is the dominant vessel (54%). The medial branch has a larger caliber in 18%, but blood flow through the perforators is lowest in these cases. According to their results, in 28%, the DIEA runs as a singular vessel with small, multiple side branches centrally at the posterior surface of the muscle. Other clinical and anatomical findings have shown that the pedicle can also divide into three branches, which happens in 14% of all cases, making it possible to split the muscle without endangering the blood supply of each segment [322, 399, 405]. Thus, perforators can penetrate the muscle laterally, medially, or at its center. The highest density of cutaneous perforators from the DIEA can be found around the umbilicus [46]. A detailed anatomical study by Blondeel et al. revealed between two and eight perforators on each side of the muscle, all with a diameter of at least 0.5 mm. Most of these vessels were located in an area 1–6 cm lateral and between 2 cm cranial and 6 cm caudal to the umbilicus [35]. Vandevoort et al. described the topography of the perforators and their course through the rectus muscle in a series of 100 clinical cases. In 65%, they found a short direct course through the muscle, whereas in 16%, the perforators pierced through a tendinous inscription. A long intramuscular course of the perforators was only found in 9%, but flap raising was most difficult in these cases [407]. Similar results were reported by Munholz et al., who found 34% of the perforators located in a lateral row along the rectus muscle, with a rectilinear course through the muscle in 79%. In the medial row, only 18.2% showed this configuration [274]. In their anatomic investigation on 329 DIEA perforators, Kikuchi et al. differentiated between "large" perforators having a diameter of at least 1 mm [140], suitable perforators that run parallel to the muscle fibers [261], and "ideal" perforators that join both features [83]. These ideal perforators were located at the intermediate third of the rectus muscle, 10–30 mm lateral to the umbilicus [185]. With a theoretical model, Patel and Keller described the arterial flow in the DIEAP flap perforators and concluded that the flap is best perfused by a single but large-diameter vessel. Although inclusion of additional perforators will increase the flow, the authors did not consider this additional trauma of dissection and increased operating time as beneficial to the patient [291]. The importance of selecting a large perforator with a palpable pulse and a diameter of at least 1 mm was stressed by Kroll, who found a high rate of fat necrosis in his first DIEAP flaps performed in unselected patients; these patients often had small perforating vessels [213]. On the other hand, it could be shown that blood flow in the perforator is higher than in the source artery and increases with time [107]. When choosing a long pedicle perforator flap, the DSEA can also be selected as the vascular pedicle instead of the DIEA. This was confirmed in an anatomical and clinical study conducted by Mah et al., who used a deep superior epigastric artery perforator flap with a long pedicle for sternal reconstruction [229].

Advantages and Disadvantages

Since its first descriptions, the DIEAP flap has proved to be a valuable and safe alternative to the conventional TRAM flap, as long as the dissection and anastomosis of the perforators can technically be mastered by the surgeon. Thus, the decision on whether to raise a conventional rectus abdominis or TRAM flap or to choose a true perforator flap with a short pedicle is mainly dependent on microsurgical skills, but apart from this, other factors also influence the type of flap to be raised. Since the main advantage of the DIEAP is the targeted dissection of the perforator and the possibility to leave the rectus muscle completely intact in patients needing guaranteed integrity of the muscular abdominal wall, the slightly higher risk of vascular complications associated with a short and small-caliber pedicle seems to be justified. Blondeel et al. reported greater venous congestion in zone IV when using the DIEAP flap compared to the conventional TRAM flap, which they explained with a dominant venous drainage of the superficial venous system within this area [37].

Therefore, if a strong superficial epigastric vein is present, they suggested performing an additional venous anastomosis. This additional venous drainage also was performed by Tran et al. in five of their 100 consecutive DIEAP flaps with favorable results [392]. Venous drainage of zones I–III is always guaranteed by the deep inferior epigastric vessels alone [37, 52]. If the comitant veins of the primary anastomosis are found to be widely thrombosed, a venous bypass using the ipsilateral basilica vein to the superficial inferior epigastric vein is possible [129]. A similar method as a solution for venous congestions can be a venous bypass to any chest wall vein, even if the primary venous anastomosis is still patent [392]. Also, a reverse-flow venous anastomosis can be established between the superficial and the deep inferior epigastric veins [223]. On the other hand, Cheng et al. found necrosis in only one out of 74 flaps in zone IV, but fat necrosis in 13.5% [66]. Using computed tomographic angiography on DIEP flaps from fresh cadavers, Schaverien et al. showed that zone IV was not perfused following injection of the lateral row perforators, so that a medial row perforator should be selected if zone IV perfusion is required [336]. As with the anterolateral thigh perforator flap, measures for preoperative imaging were proposed for planning perforator flaps. Whereas Rozen et al. used CT angiography with a good correlation between imaging and the operative findings [320], Blondeel and co-workers prefer using the color Duplex scanning method [35]. As an alternative to the commonly used horizontal design of the skin paddle, a vertical orientation of the DIEAP flap was proposed, especially in patients with midline abdominal scars, which extended up to 13 cm in length [330, 374]. To speed up flap raising and to reduce the difficulty in perforator identification, an antegrade pedicle dissection is proposed instead of the commonly used retrograde dissection, which often leads to prolonged operating time [104]. By including the sensate branch of the segmental nerve, which runs along with the perforating vessel, sensory nerve repair in perforator flaps for autologous breast reconstruction is possible. When performing a nerve anastomosis, a better response was given to pressure and thermal stimuli compared to flaps without nerve repair [36]. A critical review of perioperative complications was given by Hofer et al., who initially found a high 40% complication rate in the first 30 DIEAP flaps. As a consequence of continuous learning, perioperative complications in the next 144 flaps were reduced to 13% with only one complete flap loss [156].Donor site complications of the DIEAP flap are reported to be lower compared to the TRAM flap [31, 122, 137], but can be higher in women with preexisting scars [290]. Also in overweight or obese women undergoing breast reconstruction with the DIEAP flap, the occurrence of abdominal wall laxity, herniation, or bulging was uncommon and not statistically different from normal-weight patients [115]. On the other hand, Vyas et al. found obesity to be a significant risk factor for donor site complications, whereas in their study, no significant increase in donor site complications was associated with prior abdominal operations [411]. Bajaj et al. compared donor site-related complications between free DIEAP and muscle-sparing TRAM flaps and found no differences. Therefore, they advocated using the most expeditious and reliable flap based on the vascular anatomy of the DIEP system [16]. In a direct comparison of unilateral DIEAP versus TRAM flaps, Schaverien et al. found no differences in terms of subjective functional limitations of daily activities between both groups [337]. Abdominal strength was objectively determined after raising muscle-sparing TRAM or DIEAP flaps by Bonde and co-workers. They found a clinically small but significant advantage in the DIEAP group when measuring the eccentric muscle strength [39].

To minimize abdominal donor site morbidity, flaps based at the superficial vascular system (SIEA) were proposed instead of DIEAP perforator or muscle-sparing TRAM flaps, since harvesting flaps at the superficial inferior epigastric artery proved to be the least invasive method with no muscle injury at all [437]. Muscle injury can also be reduced if damage to motor nerves is avoided during perforator dissection. In an anatomical study, Rozen et al. found four to seven nerve branches entering the rectus muscle from the lateral border or posterior surface, running with the most lateral branch of the DIEA and its perforators. Thus, the medial row perforators, which are not related to those motor nerves, are ideal for inclusion in the flap. Using intraoperative stimulation, they also found small nerves innervating small longitudinal strips of rectus muscle, which may be sacrificed without functional detriment due to overlapping innervation from adjacent nerves. However, large nerves at the level of the arcuate line innervate the entire width of the rectus muscle and may contribute to donor-site morbidity if sacrificed [319]. The appearance of the donor site after DIEAP flap harvesting can be improved if musculofascial plication techniques and abdominoplasties are carried out immediately after flap harvesting [273].

Flap Raising

Patient Positioning

The patient is placed in the supine position and the whole abdomen is prepped across the midline, including both lower rib arches and both sides of the upper thigh as well as the pubic area. As is proposed for the other perforator flaps, the perforators can be localized around the umbilicus using Doppler before surgery to facilitate identification of a suitable perforator. This is especially the case if a small flap is planned with the perforator in the center of the skin island. Because of their constant anatomy, no preoperative diagnostic measures concerning the deep inferior epigastric vessels are necessary.

Flap Design

Because the location of the skin paddle of the DIEAP flap depends completely on the perforator selected for flap raising, the final design of the flap cannot be determined before a useful perforator showing a strong pulsation has been exposed. The most suitable perforators normally can be found at the intermediate third of the rectus muscle, 10–30 mm lateral to the umbilicus. Since the perforators feed a dense subcutaneous network of vessels, which communicate through a system of choke arteries, the skin paddle can be oriented in any direction, as long as a strong periumbilical perforator is included. To increase the safety of the flap, it should not be extended to zone IV, which means lateral to the opposite linea semilunaris. On the ipsilateral side, the skin paddle can reach up to the costal margin, if an oblique flap design is selected. This design corresponds to the dominant orientation of the subcutaneous network. Depending on the laxity of the abdominal skin and the orientation of the flap axis, the width of the flap can be 10 cm or more. The dominant orientation of the subdermal vascular network is 45° from the horizontal, and the highest density of cutaneous perforators from the deep inferior epigastric artery can be found around the umbilicus. Thus, an oblique design of the skin paddle close to the umbilicus is the most reliable.

The skin is incised down to the anterior rectus sheath, including at least one strong perforator according to the preoperative mapping using the Doppler. The medial edge of the flap is located at the midline, and the lateral flap pole can reach the costal arch.

Step 1

Starting laterally, the skin paddle is elevated at the level above the fascia, and dissection is carried out towards the semilunaris line. A few cm medially, the first perforator becomes visible, and its strength and pulse is observed.

Step 2

The dissection of the skin paddle is continued superficial to the anterior rectus sheath, and a second strong perforator is exposed close to the umbilicus. The skin paddle is completely mobilised around these two perforators.

Step 3

The skin paddle is carefully elevated, an the anterior rectus sheath is completely exposed to prepare for further dissection of the vessels. In slim patients the DIEA becomes indirectly visible by slightly lifting the flap upwards.

Step 4

The anterior rectus sheath is carefully incised around the first perforator, and the accompanying sensible nerve, if present, is transected.

Step 5

The incision of the fascia is continued to the second perforator, and the muscle fibers are bluntly separated to expose the DIEA.

Step 6

The DIEA is circumferentially dissected, and a loop is placed around the vessel. Side branches to the rectus muscle are clipped or cautherised.

Step 7

The DIEA is dissected distally without removing any muscle tissue, which only is separated bluntly. The posterior rectus sheath is left untouched.

Step 8

Step 9   According to the pedicle length needed, the DIEA is followed towards its origin from the external iliac artery without further incision of the abdominal skin.

Step 10   Cranial of the perforators, the deep inferior epigastric vessels are ligated and transected, so that the flap is now only perfused via its main distal pedicle.

Step 11   The deep inferior epigastric artery perforator flap is now ready for microvascular transfer. If needed, the flap can be thinned by removing excess fatty tissue, leaving the subdermal vascular plexus and the region around the perforators untouched. The rectus muscle is sutured, a drain is inserted, an the anterior rectus sheath is closed. Finally, the skin is approximated and sutured after mobilisation of the edges.

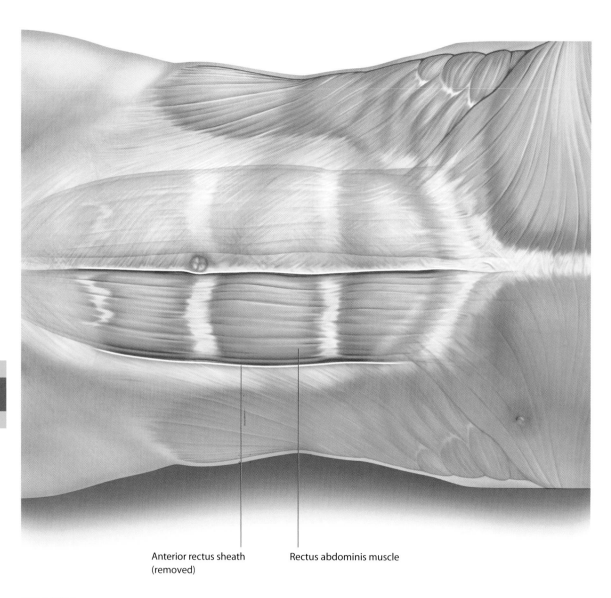

Anterior rectus sheath (removed)

Rectus abdominis muscle

Muscles of the abdomen and anterior rectus sheath

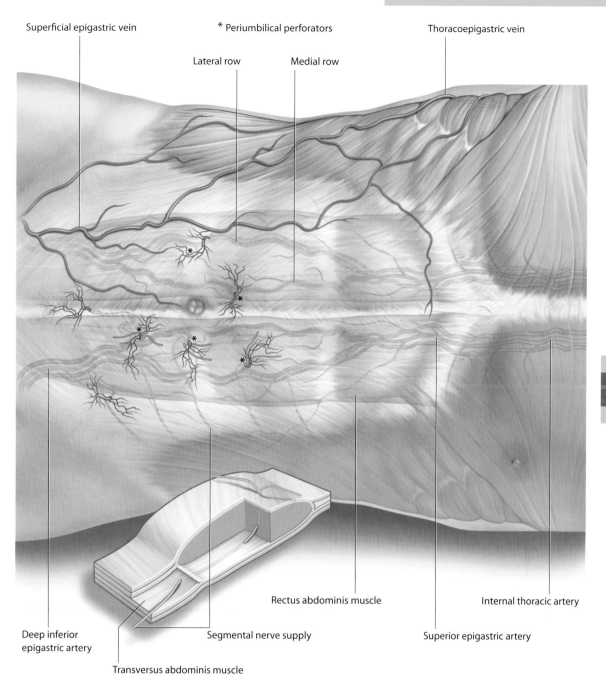

Superficial epigastric vein

* Periumbilical perforators

Thoracoepigastric vein

Lateral row

Medial row

Rectus abdominis muscle

Internal thoracic artery

Deep inferior
epigastric artery

Segmental nerve supply

Superior epigastric artery

Transversus abdominis muscle

Blood supply of the abdomen via the deep system

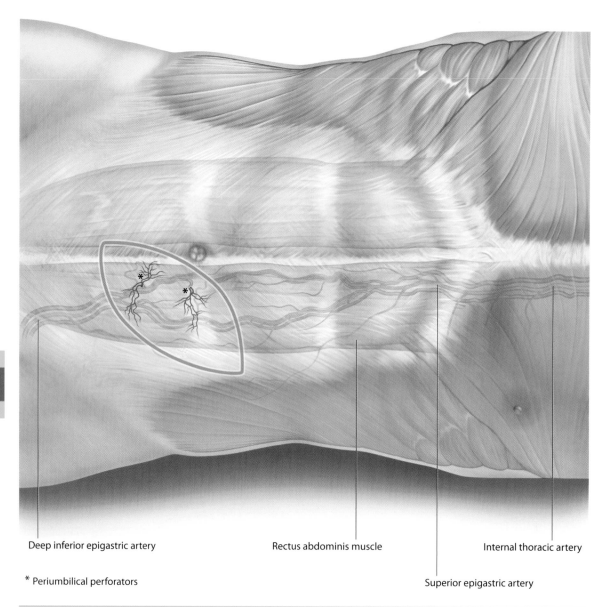

Deep inferior epigastric artery

Rectus abdominis muscle

Internal thoracic artery

* Periumbilical perforators

Superior epigastric artery

Oblique design of skin paddle close to the umbilicus is most reliable for safe blood supply

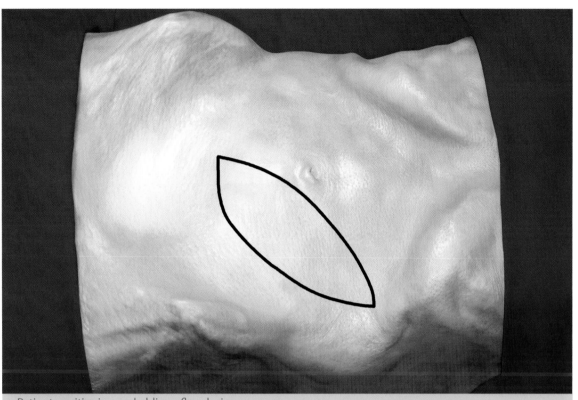

Patient positioning and oblique flap design

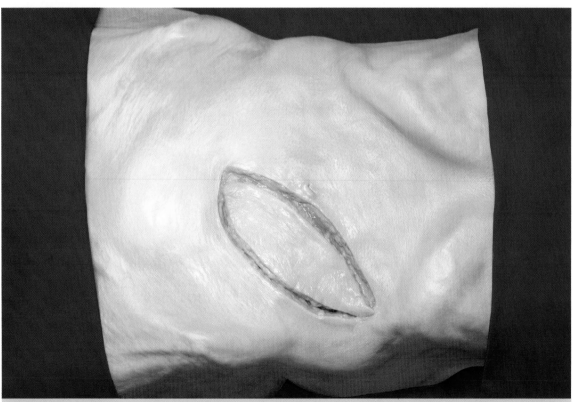

Step 1 • Incision of skin until muscle fascia

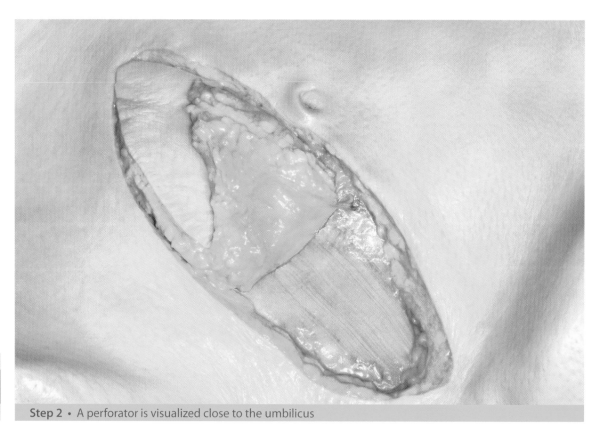

Step 2 • A perforator is visualized close to the umbilicus

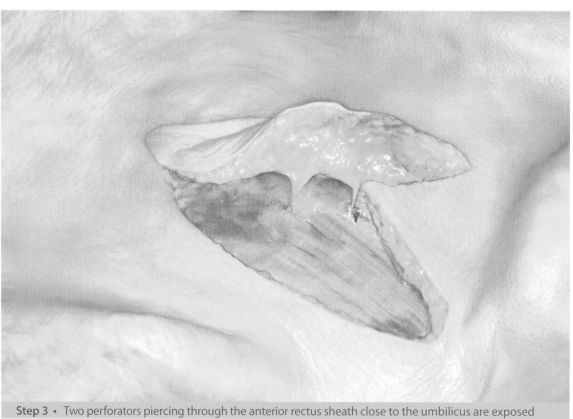

Step 3 • Two perforators piercing through the anterior rectus sheath close to the umbilicus are exposed

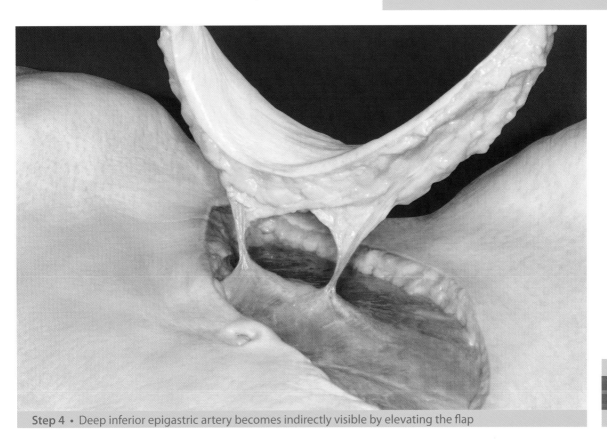

Step 4 • Deep inferior epigastric artery becomes indirectly visible by elevating the flap

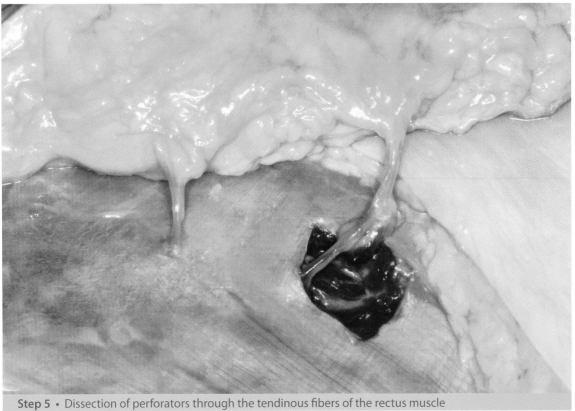

Step 5 • Dissection of perforators through the tendinous fibers of the rectus muscle

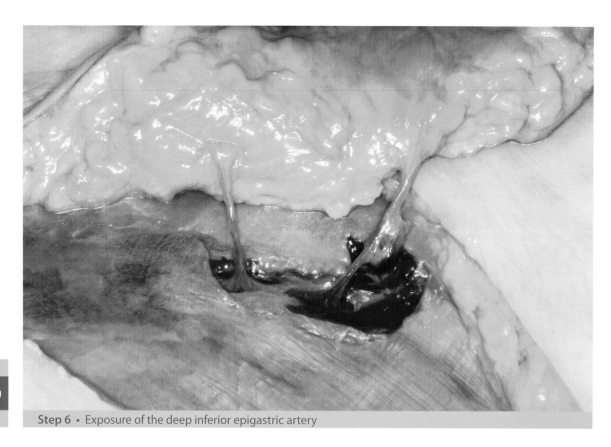

Step 6 • Exposure of the deep inferior epigastric artery

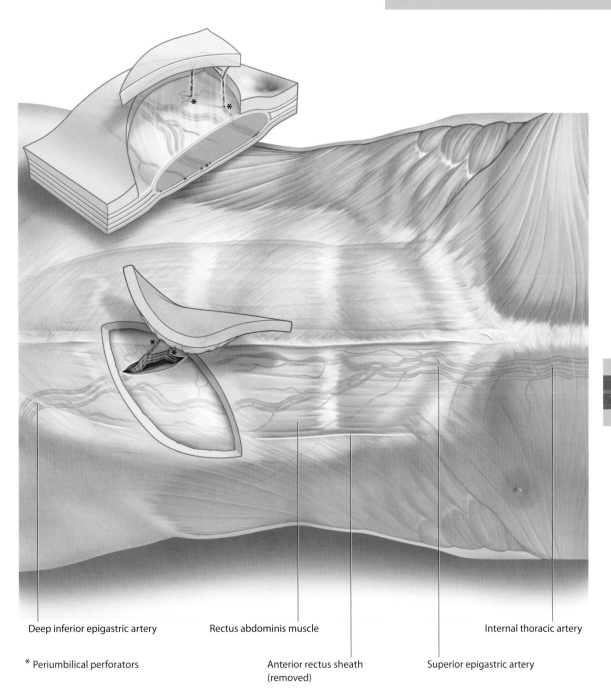

211

Deep inferior epigastric artery

Rectus abdominis muscle

Internal thoracic artery

* Periumbilical perforators

Anterior rectus sheath
(removed)

Superior epigastric artery

Perforators and their relation to the deep inferior epigastric artery

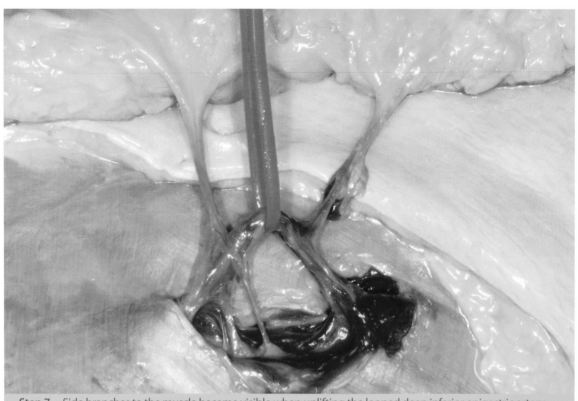

Step 7 • Side branches to the muscle become visible when uplifting the looped deep inferior epigastric artery

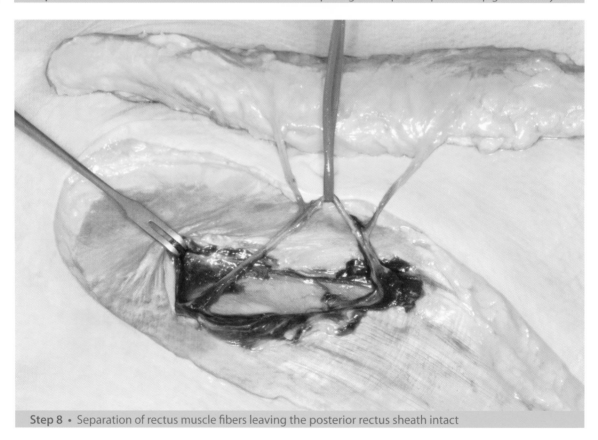

Step 8 • Separation of rectus muscle fibers leaving the posterior rectus sheath intact

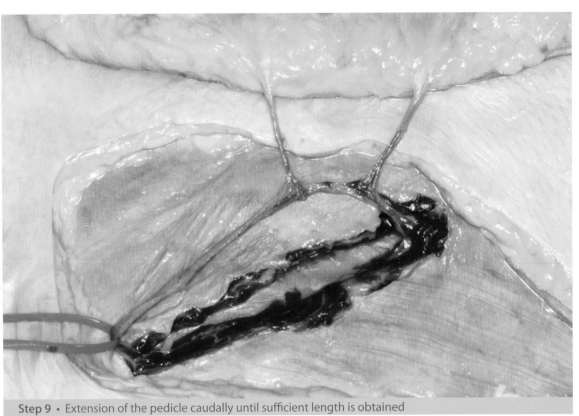

Step 9 • Extension of the pedicle caudally until sufficient length is obtained

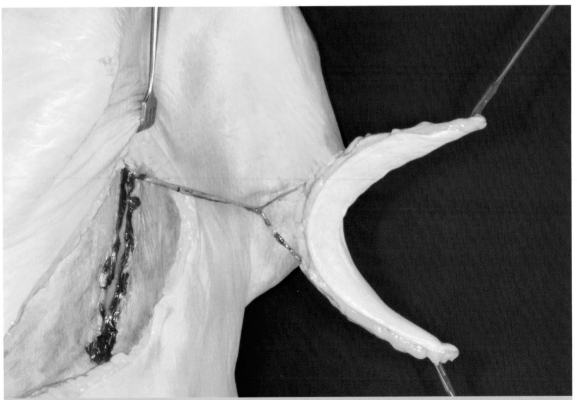

Step 10 • Ligation and transection of the deep inferior epigastric artery cranially of the second perforator

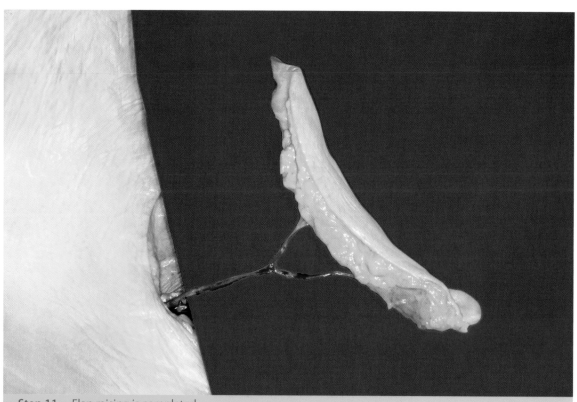

Step 11 • Flap raising is completed

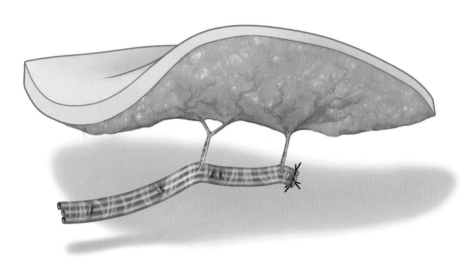

Raised deep inferior epigastric artery perforator flap after ligation toward the deep superior epigastric artery. Pedicle consisting of one artery and two veins

Comments

Flap Design

Outlining the flap is always safe when it is oblique and close to the umbilicus, where the highest density of cutaneous perforators from the deep inferior epigastric artery can be found.

Step 1: The skin island should be circumcised so that the main perforating vessels are safely included. Preoperative mapping of the main perforator using an audible Doppler can facilitate planning the flap design.

Step 2: The subcutaneous layer should be incised and dissected from lateral toward the umbilicus. This makes dissection easier and it is less likely that a perforator is missed.

Step 4: Following the perforator always leads to the deep inferior epigastric artery, so this vessel must not be searched for separately.

Step 6: Uplifting the deep inferior epigastric artery helps localize side branches, which must be carefully clipped. The posterior rectus sheath must not be opened.

Step 9: The deep inferior epigastric artery does not have to be dissected until the external iliac artery when pedicle length becomes sufficient before.

Step 10: The deep superior epigastric artery can also be used as the source vessel.

References

1. Abu Jamra FN, Afeiche N, Sumrani NB (1983) The use of a vastus lateralis muscle flap to repair a gluteal defect. Br J Plast Surg 36:319–321

2. Acland R (1972) A new needle for microvascular surgery. Surgery 71:130–131

3. Acland RD (1974) Microvascular anastomosis: a device for holding stay sutures and a new vascular clamp. Surgery 75:185–187

4. Acland RD (1979) The free iliac flap: a lateral modification of the free groin flap. Plast Reconstr Surg 64:30–36

5. Alkureishi LW, Shaw-Dunn J, Ross GL (2003) Effects of thinning the anterolateral thigh flap on the blood supply to the skin. Br J Plast Surg 56:401–408

6. Allen RJ (1998) The superior gluteal artery perforator flap. Clin Plast Surg 25:293–302

7. Allen RJ, Treece P (1994) Deep inferior epigastric perforator flap for breast reconstruction. Ann Plast Surg 32:32–38

8. Allen RJ, Kaplan J (2000) Reconstruction of a parotidectomy defect using a paraumbilical perforator flap without deep inferior epigastric vessels. J Reconstr Microsurg 16:255–257; discussion 258–259

9. Amarante J, Costa H, Reis J et al (1986) A new distally based fasciocutaneous flap of the leg. Br J Plast Surg 39:338–340

10. Anthony JP, Mathes SJ, Alpert BS (1991) The muscle flap in the treatment of chronic lower extremity osteomyelitis: results in patients over 5 years after treatment. Plast Reconstr Surg 88:311–318

11. Antia NH, Buch VI (1971) Transfer of an abdominal dermo-fat graft by direct anastomosis of blood vessels. Br J Plast Surg 24:15–19

12. Ao M, Nagase Y, Mae O et al (1997) Reconstruction of posttraumatic defects of the foot by flow-through anterolateral or anteromedial thigh flaps with preservation of posterior tibial vessels. Ann Plast Surg 38:598–603

13. Ao M, Uno K, Maeta M et al (1999) De-epithelialised anterior (anterolateral and anteromedial) thigh flaps for dead space filling and contour correction in head and neck reconstruction. Br J Plast Surg 52:261–267

14. Arnold PG, Pairolero PC (1984) Chest wall reconstruction. Experience with 100 consecutive patients. Ann Surg 199:725–732

15. Asko-Seljavaara S, Lahteenmaki T, Waris T et al (1987) Comparison of latissimus dorsi and rectus abdominis free flaps. Br J Plast Surg 40:620–628

16. Bajaj AK, Chevray PM, Chang DW (2006) Comparison of donor-site complications and functional outcomes in free muscle-sparing TRAM flap and free DIEP flap breast reconstruction. Plast Reconstr Surg 117:737–746; discussion 747–750

17. Baker SR (1981) Reconstruction of mandibular defects with the revascularized free tensor fascia lata osteomyocutaneous flap. Arch Otolaryngol 107:414–418

18. Baker SR (1984) Closure of large orbital-maxillary defects with free latissimus dorsi myocutaneous flaps. Head Neck Surg 6:828–835

19. Baker SR, Sullivan MJ (1988) Osteocutaneous free scapular flap for one-stage mandibular reconstruction. Arch Otolaryngol Head Neck Surg 114:267–277

20. Bardsley AF, Soutar DS, Elliot D et al (1990) Reducing morbidity in the radial forearm flap donor site. Plast Reconstr Surg 86:287–292; discussion 293–294

21. Bartlett SP, May JW Jr, Yaremchuk MJ (1981) The latissimus dorsi muscle: a fresh cadaver study of the primary neurovascular pedicle. Plast Reconstr Surg 67:631–636

22. Barton FE Jr, Spicer TE, Byrd HS (1983) Head and neck reconstruction with the latissimus dorsi myocutaneous flap: anatomic observations and report of 60 cases. Plast Reconstr Surg 71:199–204

23. Barwick WJ, Goodkind DJ, Serafin D (1982) The free scapular flap. Plast Reconstr Surg 69:779–787

24. Batchelor AG, Bardsley AF (1987) The bi-scapular flap. Br J Plast Surg 40:510–512

25. Bauer TR, Schoeller T, Wechselberger G et al (1999) The radial artery perforator free flap. Plast Reconstr Surg 104:885

26. Bianchi A, Doig CM, Cohen SJ (1983) The reverse latissimus dorsi flap for congenital diaphragmatic hernia repair. J Pediatr Surg 18:560–563

27. Bitter K (1980) Bone transplants from the iliac crest to the maxillo-facial region by the microsurgical technique. J Maxillofac Surg 8:210–216

218

28. Bitter K, Danai T (1983) The iliac bone or osteocutaneous transplant pedicled to the deep circumflex iliac artery. I. Anatomical and technical considerations. J Maxillofac Surg 11:195–200

29. Bitter K, Schlesinger S, Westermann U (1983) The iliac bone or osteocutaneous transplant pedicled to the deep circumflex iliac artery. II. Clinical application. J Maxillofac Surg 11:241–247

30. Black PW, Bevin AG, Arnold PG (1971) One-stage palate reconstruction with a free neo-vascularized jejunal graft. Plast Reconstr Surg 47:316–320

31. Blondeel N, Vanderstraeten GG, Monstrey SJ et al (1997) The donor site morbidity of free DIEP flaps and free TRAM flaps for breast reconstruction. Br J Plast Surg 50:322–330

32. Blondeel PN, Boeckx WD (1994) Refinements in free flap breast reconstruction: the free bilateral deep inferior epigastric perforator flap anastomosed to the internal mammary artery. Br J Plast Surg 47:495–501

33. Blondeel PN, Morrison CM (2005) Deep inferior epigastric artery perforator flap. In Blondeel PN, Hallock GG, Morris SF et al (eds) Perforator Flaps: Anatomy, Technique and Clinical Applications. Quality Medical Publishing, Inc., St. Louis, pp 385–404

34. Blondeel PN, Hallock GG, Morris SF et al (eds) (2005) Perforator Flaps: Anatomy, Technique and Clinical ApplicationsQuality Medical Publishing, Inc., St. Louis

35. Blondeel PN, Beyens G, Verhaeghe R et al (1998) Doppler flowmetry in the planning of perforator flaps. Br J Plast Surg 51:202–209

36. Blondeel PN, Demuynck M, Mete D et al (1999) Sensory nerve repair in perforator flaps for autologous breast reconstruction: sensational or senseless? Br J Plast Surg 52:37–44

37. Blondeel PN, Arnstein M, Verstraete K et al (2000) Venous congestion and blood flow in free transverse rectus abdominis myocutaneous and deep inferior epigastric perforator flaps. Plast Reconstr Surg 106:1295–1299

38. Bodde EW, de Visser E, Duysens JE et al (2003) Donor-site morbidity after free vascularized autogenous fibular transfer: subjective and quantitative analyses. Plast Reconstr Surg 111:2237–2242

39. Bonde CT, Lund H, Fridberg M et al (2007) Abdominal strength after breast reconstruction using a free abdominal flap. J Plast Reconstr Aesthet Surg 60:519–523

40. Boorman JG, Green MF (1986) A split Chinese forearm flap for simultaneous oral lining and skin cover. Br J Plast Surg 39:179–182

41. Boorman JG, Brown JA, Sykes PJ (1987) Morbidity in the forearm flap donor arm. Br J Plast Surg 40:207–212

42. Bootz F (1988) [The free forearm flap in covering defects of the pharynx and oral cavity]. HNO 36:462–6

43. Bostwick J 3rd, Vasconez LO, Jurkiewicz MJ (1978) Breast reconstruction after a radical mastectomy. Plast Reconstr Surg 61:682–693

44. Bostwick J 3rd, Nahai F, Wallace JG et al (1979) Sixty latissimus dorsi flaps. Plast Reconstr Surg 63:31–41

45. Bovet JL, Nassif TM, Guimberteau JC et al (1982) The vastus lateralis musculocutaneous flap in the repair of trochanteric pressure sores: technique and indications. Plast Reconstr Surg 69:830–834

46. Boyd JB, Taylor GI, Corlett R (1984) The vascular territories of the superior epigastric and the deep inferior epigastric systems. Plast Reconstr Surg 73:1–16

47. Brown RG, Vasconez LO, Jurkiewicz MJ (1975) Transverse abdominal flaps and the deep epigastric arcade. Plast Reconstr Surg 55:416–421

48. Bunkis J, Walton RL, Mathes SJ (1983) The rectus abdominis free flap for lower extremity reconstruction. Ann Plast Surg 11:373–380

49. Burd A, Pang P (2003) The antero-lateral thigh (ALT) flap: a pragmatic approach. Br J Plast Surg 56:837–839

50. Burns JT, Schlafly B (1986) Use of the parascapular flap in hand reconstruction. J Hand Surg Am 11:872–875

51. Carr AJ, Macdonald DA, Waterhouse N (1988) The blood supply of the osteocutaneous free fibular graft. J Bone Joint Surg Br 70:319–321

52. Carramenha e Costa MA, Carriquiry C, Vasconez LO et al (1987) An anatomic study of the venous drainage of the transverse rectus abdominis musculocutaneous flap. Plast Reconstr Surg 79:208–217

53. Carrel A (1906) The surgery of blood vessels etc. John Hopkins Hosp Bull 18:18

54. Carriquiry C, Aparecida Costa M, Vasconez LO (1985) An anatomic study of the septocutaneous vessels of the leg. Plast Reconstr Surg 76:354–363

55. Cassel JM (1989) Intramuscular anatomy of the latissimus dorsi muscle. Br J Plast Surg 42:607–609

56. Cavadas PC, Sanz-Gimenez-Rico JR, Gutierrez-de la Camara A et al (2001) The medial sural artery perforator free flap. Plast Reconstr Surg 108:1609–1615; discussion 1616–1617

57. Celik N, Wei FC, Lin CH et al (2002) Technique and strategy in anterolateral thigh perforator flap surgery, based on an analysis of 15 complete and partial failures in 439 cases. Plast Reconstr Surg 109:2211–2216; discussion 2217–2218

58. Chen D, Jupiter JB, Lipton HA et al (1989) The parascapular flap for treatment of lower extremity disorders. Plast Reconstr Surg 84:108–116

59. Chen HC, Tang YB (2003) Anterolateral thigh flap: an ideal soft tissue flap. Clin Plast Surg 30:383–401

60. Chen HC, Tang YB, Noordhoff MS (1991) Posterior tibial artery flap for reconstruction of the esophagus. Plast Reconstr Surg 88:980–986

61. Chen HC, Tang YB, Noordhoff MS (1992) Patch esophagoplasty with free forearm flap for focal stricture of the pharyngoesophageal junction and the cervical esophagus. Plast Reconstr Surg 90:45–52

62. Chen HC, Ganos DL, Coessens BC et al (1992) Free forearm flap for closure of difficult oronasal fistulas in cleft palate patients. Plast Reconstr Surg 90:757–762

63. Chen RS, Liu YX, Liu CB et al (1999) Anatomic basis of iliac crest flap pedicled on the iliolumbar artery. Surg Radiol Anat 21:103–107

64. Chen ZW, Yan W (1983) The study and clinical application of the osteocutaneous flap of fibula. Microsurgery 4:11–16

65. Cheng BS (1983) [Free forearm flap transplantation in repair and reconstruction of tongue defects]. Zhonghua Kou Qiang Ke Za Zhi 18:39–41

66. Cheng MH, Robles JA, Ulusal BG et al (2006) Reliability of zone IV in the deep inferior epigastric perforator flap: a single center's experience with 74 cases. Breast 15:158–166

67. Chicarilli ZN, Ariyan S, Glenn WW et al (1985) Management of recalcitrant bronchopleural fistulas with muscle flap obliteration. Plast Reconstr Surg 75:882–887

68. Chiu DT, Sherman JE, Edgerton BW (1984) Coverage of the calvarium with a free parascapular flap. Ann Plast Surg 12:60–66

69. Choi SW, Park JY, Hur MS et al (2007) An anatomic assessment on perforators of the lateral circumflex femoral artery for anterolateral thigh flap. J Craniofac Surg 18:866–871

70. Christ JE, Spira M (1982) Application of the latissimus dorsi muscle to the heart. Ann Plast Surg 8:118–121

71. Chuang DC, Chen HC, Wei FC et al (1992) Compound functioning free muscle flap transplantation (lateral half of soleus, fibula, and skin flap). Plast Reconstr Surg 89:335–339

72. Ciria-Llorens G, Gomez-Cia T (2001) Hand blood supply in radial forearm flap donor extremities: a qualitative analysis using doppler examination. J Hand Surg Br 26:125–128

73. Civantos FJ Jr, Burkey B, Lu FL et al (1997) Lateral arm microvascular flap in head and neck reconstruction. Arch Otolaryngol Head Neck Surg 123:830–836

74. Coghlan BA, Townsend PL (1993) The morbidity of the free vascularised fibula flap. Br J Plast Surg 46:466–469

75. Cohen BE, Cronin ED (1984) Breast reconstruction with the latissimus dorsi musculocutaneous flap. Clin Plast Surg 11:287–302

76. Coleman JJ 3rd, Sultan MR (1991) The bipedicled osteocutaneous scapula flap: a new subscapular system free flap. Plast Reconstr Surg 87:682–692

77. Coleman SC, Burkey BB, Day TA et al (2000) Increasing use of the scapula osteocutaneous free flap. Laryngoscope 110:1419–1424

78. Coleman SS, Anson BJ (1961) Arterial patterns in the hand based upon a study of 650 specimens. Surg Gynecol Obstet 113:409–424

79. Colen SR, Shaw WW, McCarthy JG (1986) Review of the morbidity of 300 free-flap donor sites. Plast Reconstr Surg 77:948–953

80. Cormack GC, Lamberty BG (1983) The anatomical vascular basis of the axillary fascio-cutaneous pedicled flap. Br J Plast Surg 36:425–427

81. Cormack GC, Lamberty BG (1984) Fasciocutaneous vessels in the upper arm: application to the design of new fasciocutaneous flaps. Plast Reconstr Surg 74:244–250

82. Culbertson JH, Mutimer K (1987) The reverse lateral upper arm flap for elbow coverage. Ann Plast Surg 18:62–68

83. D'Este S (1912) La technique de'l amputation de la mamelle pour carcinome mammarie. Revue de Chirurgie (Paris) 45:164

84. Dabb RW, Davis RM (1984) Latissimus dorsi free flaps in the elderly: an alternative to below-knee amputation. Plast Reconstr Surg 73:633–640

85. Daniel RK (1978) Mandibular reconstruction with free tissue transfers. Ann Plast Surg 1:346–371

86. Daniel RK, Taylor GI (1973) Distant transfer of an island flap by microvascular anastomoses. A clinical technique. Plast Reconstr Surg 52:111–117

87. Daniel RK, Williams HB (1973) The free transfer of skin flaps by microvascular anastomoses. An experimental study and a reappraisal. Plast Reconstr Surg 52:16–31

88. Deiler S, Pfadenhauer A, Widmann J et al (2000) Tensor fasciae latae perforator flap for reconstruction of composite Achilles tendon defects with skin and vascularized fascia. Plast Reconstr Surg 106:342–349

89. Demirkan F, Chen HC, Wei FC et al (2000) The versatile anterolateral thigh flap: a musculocutaneous flap in disguise in head and neck reconstruction. Br J Plast Surg 53:30–36

90. Deraemacher R, Thienen CV, Lejour M et al (1988) The serratus anterior-scapular free flaps: A new osteomuscular unit for reconstruction after radical head and neck surgery (abstract) Proceedings of the Second International Conference of Head and Neck Cancer.

91. Disa JJ, Cordeiro PG (1998) The current role of preoperative arteriography in free fibula flaps. Plast Reconstr Surg 102:1083–1088

92. dos Santos LF (1980) The scapular flap: a new microsurgical free flap. Bol Chir Plast 70:133

93. dos Santos LF (1984) The vascular anatomy and dissection of the free scapular flap. Plast Reconstr Surg 73:599–604

94. Dowden RV, McCraw JB (1980) The vastus lateralis muscle flap: technique and applications. Ann Plast Surg 4:396–404

95. Drever JM, Hodson-Walker N (1985) Closure of the donor defect for breast reconstruction with rectus abdominis myocutaneous flaps. Plast Reconstr Surg 76:558–565

96. Drimmer MA, Krasna MJ (1987) The vastus lateralis myocutaneous flap. Plast Reconstr Surg 79:560–566

97. Ebihara H, Maruyama Y (1989) Free abdominal flaps: variations in design and application to soft tissue defects of the head. J Reconstr Microsurg 5:193–201

98. Ehrenfeld M (1990) Korrektur subcutaner Weichgewebsdefekte durch mikrochirurgische Transplantate. In: Schuchardt K (ed) Fortschritte der Kiefer- und Gesichtschirurgie. Thieme, Stuttgart

99. Ehrenfeld M, Cornelius CP, Rossell L (1992) Microvascular bone transplantation. Developments and present concept. J Craniomaxillofac Surg 20:35–67

221

100. Elliot D, Bardsley AF, Batchelor AG et al (1988) Direct closure of the radial forearm flap donor defect. Br J Plast Surg 41:358–360

101. Emerson DJ, Sprigg A, Page RE (1985) Some observations on the radial artery island flap. Br J Plast Surg 38:107–112

102. Fassio E, Ugurlu K, Goga D et al (1999) Reconstruction of a mandibular and maxillary defect with a biscapular bifascial flap as a single transplant. J Oral Maxillofac Surg 57:1134–1137

103. Feinendegen DL, Klos D (2002) A subcostal artery perforator flap for a lumbar defect. Plast Reconstr Surg 109:2446–2449

104. Feingold RS (2009) Improving surgeon confidence in the DIEP flap: a strategy for reducing operative time with minimally invasive donor site. Ann Plast Surg 62:533–537

105. Fenton OM, Roberts JO (1985) Improving the donor site of the radial forearm flap. Br J Plast Surg 38:504–505

106. Ferreira MC, Rocha DL, Besteiro JM et al (1985) Mandibular reconstruction with free osteocutaneous iliac crest based on the deep circumflex vessels. Chir Plastica 8:83

107. Figus A, Ramakrishnan V, Rubino C (2008) Hemodynamic changes in the microcirculation of DIEP flaps. Ann Plast Surg 60:644–648

108. Fisher J, Bostwick J 3rd, Powell RW (1983) Latissimus dorsi blood supply after thoracodorsal vessel division: the serratus collateral. Plast Reconstr Surg 72:502–511

109. Fissette J, Lahaye T, Colot G (1983) The use of the free parascapular flap in midpalmar soft tissue defect. Ann Plast Surg 10:235–238

110. Flemming AF, Brough MD, Evans ND et al (1990) Mandibular reconstruction using vascularised fibula. Br J Plast Surg 43:403–409

111. Forrest C, Boyd B, Manktelow R et al (1992) The free vascularised iliac crest tissue transfer: donor site complications associated with eighty-two cases. Br J Plast Surg 45:89–93

112. Frick A, Baumeister RG, Wiebecke B (1987) [Vascular ultrastructure of the scapular flap]. Handchir Mikrochir Plast Chir 19:336–338

113. Gahhos FN, Tross RB, Salomon JC (1985) Scapular free-flap dissection made easier. Plast Reconstr Surg 75:115–118

114. Gardener E, Gray DJ, O'Rahilly R (1966) Anatomy, 3 edn. WB Saunders Co., Philadelphia

115. Garvey PB, Buchel EW, Pockaj BA et al (2005) The deep inferior epigastric perforator flap for breast reconstruction in overweight and obese patients. Plast Reconstr Surg 115:447–457

116. Geddes CR, Tang M, Yang D et al (2005) Anatomy of the Integument of the Trunk. In Blondeel PN, Hallock GG, Morris SF et al (eds) Perforator Flaps: Anatomy, Technique and Clinical Applications. Quality Medical Publishing, Inc., St. Louis, pp 359–384

117. Gedebou TM, Wei FC, Lin CH (2002) Clinical experience of 1284 free anterolateral thigh flaps. Handchir Mikrochir Plast Chir 34:239–244

118. Gegenbaur C (1888) Lehrbuch der Anatomie des Menschen, 3rd edn. V. Wilhelm Engelmann, Leipzig

119. Gehrking E, Remmert S, Majocco A (1998) [Topographic and anatomic study of lateral upper arm transplants]. Ann Anat 180:275–280

120. Gilbert A (1981) Free vascularized bone grafts. Int Surg 66:27–31

121. Gilbert A, Teot L (1982) The free scapular flap. Plast Reconstr Surg 69:601–604

122. Gill PS, Hunt JP, Guerra AB et al (2004) A 10-year retrospective review of 758 DIEP flaps for breast reconstruction. Plast Reconstr Surg 113:1153–1160

123. Godina M (1982) Discussion: the free scapular flap. Br J Plast Surg 69:786

124. Goodacre TE, Walker CJ, Jawad AS et al (1990) Donor site morbidity following osteocutaneous free fibula transfer. Br J Plast Surg 43:410–412

125. Gordon L, Buncke HJ, Alpert BS (1982) Free latissimus dorsi muscle flap with split-thickness skin graft cover: a report of 16 cases. Plast Reconstr Surg 70:173–178

126. Gravvanis A, Lo S, Shirley R (2009) Aesthetic restoration of Poland's syndrome in a male patient using free anterolateral thigh perforator flap as autologous filler. Microsurgery 29:490–494

127. Gruber W (1878) Hohe Teilung der A. poplitea in die A. tibialis postica und in den Truncus communis für die A. peronea und die A. tibialis antica, mit Endigung der A. tibialis postica als A. plantaris interna und der A. peronea als A. plantaris externa. Arch Pathol Anat Physiol Klin Med 74:438

128. Guthrie CC (1908) Some physiological aspects of blood vessel surgery. JAMA 51:1658

129. Guzzetti T, Thione A (2008) The basilic vein: an alternative drainage of DIEP flap in severe venous congestion. Microsurgery 28:555–558

130. Ha B, Baek CH (1999) Head and neck reconstruction using lateral thigh free flap: flap design. Microsurgery 19:157–165

131. Hallock GG (1988) Refinement of the radial forearm flap donor site using skin expansion. Plast Reconstr Surg 81:21–25

132. Hallock GG (1990) Cutaneous cover for cutaneous coverage. Contemp Orthop 21:234

133. Hallock GG (1991) Complications of 100 consecutive local fasciocutaneous flaps. Plast Reconstr Surg 88:264–268

134. Hallock GG (1994) Evaluation of fasciocutaneous perforators using color duplex imaging. Plast Reconstr Surg 94:644–651

135. Hallock GG (1999) The anatomy of the extended peroneal venous system. Plast Reconstr Surg 104:976–983

136. Hallock GG (2005) The superior epigastric(RECTUS ABDOMINIS) muscle perforator flap. Ann Plast Surg 55:430–432

137. Hamdi M, Weiler-Mithoff EM, Webster MH (1999) Deep inferior epigastric perforator flap in breast reconstruction: experience with the first 50 flaps. Plast Reconstr Surg 103:86–95

138. Hamilton SG, Morrison WA (1982) The scapular free flap. Br J Plast Surg 35:2–7

139. Harii K (1988) Refined microneurovascular free muscle transplantation for reanimation of paralyzed face. Microsurgery 9:169–176

140. Harii K, Ohmori K, Sekiguchi J (1976) The free musculocutaneous flap. Plast Reconstr Surg 57:294–303

141. Harii K, Ebihara S, Ono I et al (1985) Pharyngoesophageal reconstruction using a fabricated forearm free flap. Plast Reconstr Surg 75:463–476

142. Harrison DH (1986) The osteocutaneous free fibular graft. J Bone Joint Surg Br 68:804–807

143. Hartrampf CR Jr (1984) Abdominal wall competence in transverse abdominal island flap operations. Ann Plast Surg 12:139–146

144. Hatoko M, Harashina T, Inoue T et al (1990) Reconstruction of palate with radial forearm flap; a report of 3 cases. Br J Plast Surg 43:350–354

145. Hauben DJ, Smith AR, Sonneveld GJ et al (1983) The use of the vastus lateralis musculocutaneous flap for the repair of trochanteric pressure sores. Ann Plast Surg 10:359–363

146. Hayashi A, Maruyama Y (1989) The "reduced" latissimus dorsi musculocutaneous flap. Plast Reconstr Surg 84:290–295

147. Hayden R, O'Leary M (1991) A neurosensory fibula flap: Anatomical description and clinical applications. 94th Annual Meeting of the American Laryngological, Rhinological and Otological Society. Hawaii

148. Heitmann C, Khan FN, Levin LS (2003) Vasculature of the peroneal artery: an anatomic study focused on the perforator vessels. J Reconstr Microsurg 19:157–162

149. Heitmann C, Felmerer G, Durmus C et al (2000) Anatomical features of perforator blood vessels in the deep inferior epigastric perforator flap. Br J Plast Surg 53:205–208

150. Heller F, Hsu CM, Chuang CC et al (2004) Anterolateral thigh fasciocutaneous flap for simultaneous reconstruction of refractory scalp and dural defects. Report of two cases. J Neurosurg 100:1094–1097

151. Henle J (1868) Handbuch der systemischen Anatomie des Menschen. Friedrich Vieweg und Sohn. Braunschweig

152. Hidalgo DA (1989) Fibula free flap: a new method of mandible reconstruction. Plast Reconstr Surg 84:71–79

153. Hidalgo DA (1994) Fibula free flap mandible reconstruction. Microsurgery 15:238–244

154. Hidalgo DA, Carrasquillo IM (1992) The treatment of lower extremity sarcomas with wide excision, radiotherapy, and free-flap reconstruction. Plast Reconstr Surg 89:96–101; discussion 102

155. Hirase Y, Kojima T, Kinoshita Y et al (1991) Composite reconstruction for chest wall and scalp using multiple ribs-latissimus dorsi osteomyocutaneous flaps as pedicled and free flaps. Plast Reconstr Surg 87:555–561

156. Hofer SO, Damen TH, Mureau MA et al (2007) A critical review of perioperative complications in 175 free deep inferior epigastric perforator flap breast reconstructions. Ann Plast Surg 59:137–142

157. Holm C, Mayr M, Hofter E et al (2006) Perfusion zones of the DIEP flap revisited: a clinical study. Plast Reconstr Surg 117:37–43

158. Holmberg J, Ekerot L (1986) The free scapular flap. An alternative to conventional flaps on the upper extremity. Scand J Plast Reconstr Surg 20:219–223

159. Hölzle F, Hohlweg-Majert B, Kesting MR et al (2009) Reverse flow facial artery as recipient vessel for perforator flaps. Microsurgery 29:437–442

160. Howaldt HP, Bitter K (1990) Totaler Zungenersatz durch ein mikrochirurgisches Latissimus-dorsi-Transplantat. In Schuchardt K (ed) Fortschritt der Kiefer- und Gesichtschirurgie. Thieme, Stuttgart

161. Hsieh CH, Yang CC, Kuo YR et al (2003) Free anterolateral thigh adipofascial perforator flap. Plast Reconstr Surg 112:976–982

162. Huang GK, Liu ZZ, Shen YL et al (1980) Microvascular free transfer of iliac bone based on the deep circumflex iliac vessels. J Microsurg 2:113–120

163. Huang GK, Hu RQ, Miao H et al (1985) Microvascular free transfer of iliac bone based on the deep superior branches of the superior gluteal vessels. Plast Reconstr Surg 75:68–74

164. Huber GC (1930) Piersol's Human Anatomy, 9th edn. L.B. Lippincott, Philadelphia

165. Hung LK, Lao J, Ho PC (1996) Free posterior tibial perforator flap: anatomy and a report of 6 cases. Microsurgery 17:503–511

166. Huo R, Li S, Li Y et al (2002) [Microvascular structure of the transmidline scapular flap]. Zhonghua Zheng Xing Wai Ke Za Zhi 18:357–359

167. Hyrtl J (1887) Lehrbuch der Anatomie des Menschen, 19th edn. Wilhelm Braunmüller, Vienna

168. Ichinose A, Tahara S, Terashi H et al (2003) Short-term postoperative flow changes after free radial forearm flap transfer: possible cause of vascular occlusion. Ann Plast Surg 50:160–164

169. Ichinose A, Tahara S, Terashi H et al (2003) Importance of the deep vein in the drainage of a radial forearm flap: a haemodynamic study. Scand J Plast Reconstr Surg Hand Surg 37:145–149

170. Iida H, Ohashi I, Kishimoto S et al (2003) Preoperative assessment of anterolateral thigh flap cutaneous perforators by colour Doppler flowmetry. Br J Plast Surg 56:21–25

171. Inoue T, Fujino T (1986) An upper arm flap, pedicled on the cephalic vein with arterial anastomosis, for head and neck reconstruction. Br J Plast Surg 39:451–453

172. Iriarte-Ortabe J, Reycher H (1992) Mandibular reconstruction with fibular free flap. J Craniomaxillofac Surg 20:36

173. Jackson CM (1933) Morris' Human Anatomy, 9 edn. P. Blackiston's Son & Co., Inc., Philadelphia

174. Jacobson HT, Suarez EL (1960) Microsurgery in anastomosis of small vessels. Surg Forum 11

175. Ji Y, Li T, Shamburger S et al (2002) Microsurgical anterolateral thigh fasciocutaneous flap for facial contour correction in patients with hemifacial microsomia. Microsurgery 22:34–38

176. Jin YT, Guan WX, Shi TM et al (1985) Reversed island forearm fascial flap in hand surgery. Ann Plast Surg 15:340–347

177. Jones NF, Swartz WM, Mears DC et al (1988) The "double barrel" free vascularized fibular bone graft. Plast Reconstr Surg 81:378–385

178. Karcher H, Borbely L (1988) [Possibilities of vital bone grafts in the maxillofacial area]. Dtsch Z Mund Kiefer Gesichtschir 12:124–134

179. Kärcher H (1986) Die Unterkieferrekonstruktion mit freien mikrovaskulären Knochentransplantaten. Acta Chir Australiaca 33:251

180. Katsaros J, Schusterman M, Beppu M et al (1984) The lateral upper arm flap: anatomy and clinical applications. Ann Plast Surg 12:489–500

181. Kaufman T, Hurwitz DJ, Boehnke M et al (1985) The microcirculatory pattern of the transverse-abdominal flap: a cross-sectional xerographic and CAT scanning study. Ann Plast Surg 14:340–345

182. Kawamura K, Yajima H, Kobata Y et al (2005) Clinical applications of free soleus and peroneal perforator flaps. Plast Reconstr Surg 115:114–119

183. Kerawala CJ, Martin IC (2003) Palmar arch backflow following radial forearm free flap harvest. Br J Oral Maxillofac Surg 41:157–160

184. Khan UD, Miller JG (2007) Reliability of handheld Doppler in planning local perforator-based flaps for extremities. Aesthetic Plast Surg 31:521–525

185. Kikuchi N, Murakami G, Kashiwa H et al (2001) Morphometrical study of the arterial perforators of the deep inferior epigastric perforator flap. Surg Radiol Anat 23:375–381

186. Kim DY, Jeong EC, Kim KS et al (2002) Thinning of the thoracodorsal perforator-based cutaneous flap for axillary burn scar contracture. Plast Reconstr Surg 109:1372–1377

187. Kim JT (2005) New nomenclature concept of perforator flap. Br J Plast Surg 58:431–440

188. Kim JT, Koo BS, Kim SK (2001) The thin latissimus dorsi perforator-based free flap for resurfacing. Plast Reconstr Surg 107:374–382

189. Kimata Y (2003) Deep circumflex iliac perforator flap. Clin Plast Surg 30:433–438

190. Kimata Y, Uchiyama K, Ebihara S et al (1998) Anatomic variations and technical problems of the anterolateral thigh flap: a report of 74 cases. Plast Reconstr Surg 102:1517–1523

191. Kimata Y, Uchiyama K, Sekido M et al (1999) Anterolateral thigh flap for abdominal wall reconstruction. Plast Reconstr Surg 103:1191–1197

192. Kimata Y, Uchiyama K, Ebihara S et al (2000) Anterolateral thigh flap donor-site complications and morbidity. Plast Reconstr Surg 106:584–589

193. Kimura N (2002) A microdissected thin tensor fasciae latae perforator flap. Plast Reconstr Surg 109:69–77; discussion 78–80

194. Kimura N, Satoh K (1996) Consideration of a thin flap as an entity and clinical applications of the thin anterolateral thigh flap. Plast Reconstr Surg 97:985–992

195. Kimura N, Satoh K, Hasumi T et al (2001) Clinical application of the free thin anterolateral thigh flap in 31 consecutive patients. Plast Reconstr Surg 108:1197–1208; discussion 1209–1210

196. Kincaid SB (1984) Breast reconstruction: a review. Ann Plast Surg 12:431–448

197. Kleinert HE, Kasdan ML (1963) Salvage of devascularized upper extremities including studies of small vessels anastomosis. Clin Orthop Relat Res 29:29

198. Kolker AR, Coombs CJ, Meara JG (2000) A method for minimizing donor site complications of the radial forearm flap. Ann Plast Surg 45:329–331

199. Koshima I, Soeda S (1985) Repair of a wide defect of the lower leg with the combined scapular and parascapular flap. Br J Plast Surg 38:518–521

200. Koshima I, Soeda S (1989) Inferior epigastric artery skin flaps without rectus abdominis muscle. Br J Plast Surg 42:645–648

225

201. Koshima I, Soeda S (1991) Free posterior tibial perforator-based flaps. Ann Plast Surg 26:284–288

202. Koshima I, Fukuda H, Utunomiya R et al (1989) The anterolateral thigh flap; variations in its vascular pedicle. Br J Plast Surg 42:260–262

203. Koshima I, Inagawa K, Urushibara K et al (1998) Paraumbilical perforator flap without deep inferior epigastric vessels. Plast Reconstr Surg 102:1052–1057

204. Koshima I, Urushibara K, Inagawa K et al (2001) Free tensor fasciae latae perforator flap for the reconstruction of defects in the extremities. Plast Reconstr Surg 107:1759–1765

205. Koshima I, Moriguchi T, Soeda S et al (1992) Free thin paraumbilical perforator-based flaps. Ann Plast Surg 29:12–17

206. Koshima I, Yamamoto H, Moriguchi T et al (1994) Combined anteroposterior tibial perforator-based flap with a vascularized deep peroneal nerve for repair of facial defect. Ann Plast Surg 33:421–425

207. Koshima I, Hosoda M, Inagawa K et al (1996) Free medial thigh perforator-based flaps: new definition of the pedicle vessels and versatile application. Ann Plast Surg 37:507–515

208. Koshima I, Moriguchi T, Ohta S et al (1992) The vasculature and clinical application of the posterior tibial perforator-based flap. Plast Reconstr Surg 90:643–649

209. Koshima I, Yamamoto H, Hosoda M et al (1993) Free combined composite flaps using the lateral circumflex femoral system for repair of massive defects of the head and neck regions: an introduction to the chimeric flap principle. Plast Reconstr Surg 92:411–420

210. Koshima I, Kawada S, Etoh H et al (1995) Flow-through anterior thigh flaps for one-stage reconstruction of soft-tissue defects and revascularization of ischemic extremities. Plast Reconstr Surg 95:252–260

211. Koshima I, Saisho H, Kawada S et al (1999) Flow-through thin latissimus dorsi perforator flap for repair of soft-tissue defects in the legs. Plast Reconstr Surg 103:1483–1490

212. Krishna BV, Green MF (1980) Extended role of latissimus dorsi myocutaneous flap in reconstruction of the neck. Br J Plast Surg 33:233–236

213. Kroll SS (2000) Fat necrosis in free transverse rectus abdominis myocutaneous and deep inferior epigastric perforator flaps. Plast Reconstr Surg 106:576–583

214. Kuek LB, Chuan TL (1991) The extended lateral arm flap: a new modification. J Reconstr Microsurg 7:167–173

215. Kuo YR, Seng-Feng J, Kuo FM et al (2002) Versatility of the free anterolateral thigh flap for reconstruction of soft-tissue defects: review of 140 cases. Ann Plast Surg 48:161–166

216. Laitung JK, Peck F (1985) Shoulder function following the loss of the latissimus dorsi muscle. Br J Plast Surg 38:375–379

217. Lamberty BG, Cormack GC (1990) Fasciocutaneous flaps. Clin Plast Surg 17:713–726

218. Landra AP (1979) The latissimus dorsi musculocutaneous flap used to resurface a defect on the upper arm and restore extension to the elbow. Br J Plast Surg 32:275–277

219. Latarjet A (1948) Testut's traite d'anatomie humaine. 9th edn. G. Doin & Cie, Paris

220. Lee EH, Goh JC, Helm R et al (1990) Donor site morbidity following resection of the fibula. J Bone Joint Surg Br 72:129–131

221. Lejour M, Dome M (1991) Abdominal wall function after rectus abdominis transfer. Plast Reconstr Surg 87:1054–1068

222. Lin SD, Lai CS, Chiu CC (1984) Venous drainage in the reverse forearm flap. Plast Reconstr Surg 74:508–512

223. Liu TS, Ashjian P, Festekjian J (2007) Salvage of congested deep inferior epigastric perforator flap with a reverse flow venous anastomosis. Ann Plast Surg 59:214–217

224. Logan AM, Black MJ (1985) Injury to the brachial plexus resulting from shoulder positioning during latissimus dorsi flap pedicle dissection. Br J Plast Surg 38:380–382

226

225. Lorenz RR, Esclamado R (2001) Preoperative magnetic resonance angiography in fibular-free flap reconstruction of head and neck defects. Head Neck 23:844–850

226. Lovie MJ, Duncan GM, Glasson DW (1984) The ulnar artery forearm free flap. Br J Plast Surg 37:486–492

227. Lyberg T, Olstad OA (1991) The vascularized fibular flap for mandibular reconstruction. J Craniomaxillofac Surg 19:113–118

228. MacKinnon SE, Weiland AJ, Godina M (1983) Immediate forearm reconstruction with a functional latissimus dorsi island pedicle myocutaneous flap. Plast Reconstr Surg 71:706–710

229. Mah E, Rozen WM, Ashton MW et al (2009) Deep superior epigastric artery perforators: anatomical study and clinical application in sternal reconstruction. Plast Reconstr Surg 123:1719–1723

230. Malhotra K, Lian TS, Chakradeo V (2008) Vascular anatomy of anterolateral thigh flap. Laryngoscope 118:589–592

231. Malt RA, McKhann C (1964) Replantation of Several Arms. JAMA 189:716–722

232. Manchot C (1889) Die Hautarterien des menschlichen Körpers. Vogel, Leipzig

233. Manktelow RT (1986) Microvascular reconstruction. Springer-Verlag, Berlin Heidelberg, New York

234. Mao C, Cai Z, Peng X et al (2002) [The value of preoperative routine donor leg angiography in free fibula flaps]. Zhonghua Kou Qiang Yi Xue Za Zhi 37:15–17

235. Mardini S, Tsai FC, Wei FC (2003) The thigh as a model for free style free flaps. Clin Plast Surg 30:473–480

236. Mardini S, Lin CH, Wei FC (2005) Lateral circumflex femoral artery–vastus lateralis perforator flap. In Blondeel PN, Hallock GG, Morris SF et al (eds) Perforator Flaps: Anatomy, Technique and Clinical Applications. Quality Medical Publishing, Inc., St. Louis, pp 617–634

237. Maros T (1981) Data regarding the typology and functional significance of the venous valves. Morphol Embryol (Bucur) 27:195–214

238. Martin-Granizo R, Gomez F, Sanchez-Cuellar A (2002) An unusual anomaly of the radial artery with potential significance to the forearm free flap. Case report. J Craniomaxillofac Surg 30:189–191

239. Martin IC, Brown AE (1994) Free vascularized fascial flap in oral cavity reconstruction. Head Neck 16:45–50

240. Maruyama Y, Urita Y, Ohnishi K (1985) Rib-latissimus dorsi osteomyocutaneous flap in reconstruction of a mandibular defect. Br J Plast Surg 38:234–237

241. Maruyama Y, Iwahira Y, Hashimura C et al (1986) One stage total cheek reconstruction with double folded extended latissimus dorsi musculocutaneous flap. Acta Chir Plast 28:159–166

242. Masser MR (1990) The preexpanded radial free flap. Plast Reconstr Surg 86:295–301; discussion 302–303

243. Mast BA (2001) Comparison of magnetic resonance angiography and digital subtraction angiography for visualization of lower extremity arteries. Ann Plast Surg 46:261–264

244. Masuoka T, Sugita A, Sekiya S et al (2002) Breast reconstruction with perforator-based inframammary de-epithelized flap: a case report. Aesthetic Plast Surg 26:211–214

245. Mathes SJ, Nahai F (1979) Clinical atlas of muscle and musculocutaneous flaps. CV Mosby, St. Louis

246. Mathes SJ, Nahai F (1981) Classification of the vascular anatomy of muscles: experimental and clinical correlation. Plast Reconstr Surg 67:177–187

247. Mathes SJ, Nahai F (1982) Clinical applications for muscle and myocutaneous flaps. CV Mosby, St. Louis

248. Matloub HS, Larson DL, Kuhn JC et al (1989) Lateral arm free flap in oral cavity reconstruction: a functional evaluation. Head Neck 11:205–211

249. Maxwell GP, Stueber K, Hoopes JE (1978) A free latissimus dorsi myocutaneous flap: case report. Plast Reconstr Surg 62:462–466

250. Maxwell GP, Manson PN, Hoopes JE (1979) Experience with thirteen latissimus dorsi myocutaneous free flaps. Plast Reconstr Surg 64:1–8

251. Mayou BJ, Whitby D, Jones BM (1982) The scapular flap – an anatomical and clinical study. Br J Plast Surg 35:8–13

252. McCormack LJ, Cauldwell EW, Anson BJ (1953) Brachial and antebrachial arterial patterns; a study of 750 extremities. Surg Gynecol Obstet 96:43–54

253. McCraw JB, Penix JO, Baker JW (1978) Repair of major defects of the chest wall and spine with the latissimus dorsi myocutaneous flap. Plast Reconstr Surg 62:197–206

254. McGregor AD (1987) The free radial forearm flap – the management of the secondary defect. Br J Plast Surg 40:83–85

255. McGregor IA, Morgan G (1973) Axial and random pattern flaps. Br J Plast Surg 26:202–213

256. McLean DH, Buncke HJ Jr (1972) Autotransplant of omentum to a large scalp defect, with microsurgical revascularization. Plast Reconstr Surg 49:268–274

257. Meagher PJ, Morrison WA (2002) Free fibula flap-donor-site morbidity: case report and review of the literature. J Reconstr Microsurg 18:465–468; discussion 469–470

258. Meland NB, Maki S, Chao EY et al (1992) The radial forearm flap: a biomechanical study of donor-site morbidity utilizing sheep tibia. Plast Reconstr Surg 90:763–773

259. Meland NB, Fisher J, Irons GB et al (1989) Experience with 80 rectus abdominis free-tissue transfers. Plast Reconstr Surg 83:481–487

260. Mendelson BC, Masson JK (1977) Treatment of chronic radiation injury over the shoulder with a latissimus dorsi myocutaneous flap. Plast Reconstr Surg 60:681–691

261. Mendelson BC, Masson JK, Arnold PG et al (1979) Flaps used for nasal reconstruction: a perspective based on 180 cases. Mayo Clin Proc 54:91–96

262. Milloy FJ, Anson BJ, McAfee DK (1960) The rectus abdominis muscle and the epigastric arteries. Surg Gynecol Obstet 110:293–302

263. Minami RT, Hentz VR, Vistnes LM (1977) Use of vastus lateralis muscle flap for repair of trochanteric pressure sores. Plast Reconstr Surg 60:364–368

264. Miyamoto Y, Harada K, Kodama Y et al (1986) Cranial coverage involving scalp, bone and dura using free inferior epigastric flap. Br J Plast Surg 39:483–490

265. Moffett TR, Madison SA, Derr JW Jr et al (1992) An extended approach for the vascular pedicle of the lateral arm free flap. Plast Reconstr Surg 89:259–267

266. Morris H, Anson BJ (1966) Human anatomy: a complete systematic treatise, 12th edn. Blakiston Division, New York,

267. Morrison WA, Shen TY (1987) Anterior tibial artery flap: anatomy and case report. Br J Plast Surg 40:230–235

268. Morrison WA, O'Brien BM, MacLeod AM (1984) Experience with thumb reconstruction. J Hand Surg Br 9:223–233

269. Mühling J, Reuther J (1990) Indikationen zum Transfer des Latissimus-dorsi-Myokutanlappens zur Rekonstruktion im Kopf-Hals-Bereich. In Schuchardt K (ed) Fortschritte in der Kiefer- und Gesichtschirurgie. Thieme, Stuttgart

270. Muhlbauer W, Olbrisch RR (1977) The latissimus dorsi myocutaneous flap for breast reconstruction. Chir Plast 4:27–434

271. Mühlbauer W, Herndl E, Stock W (1982) The forearm flap. Plast Reconstr Surg 70:336–344

272. Mühlbauer W, Olbrisch RR, Herndl E et al (1981) [Treatment of neck contracture after burns with a free under arm flap]. Chirurg 52:635–637

273. Munhoz AM, Sturtz G, Montag E et al (2005) Clinical outcome of abdominal wall after DIEP flap harvesting and immediate application of abdominoplasty techniques. Plast Reconstr Surg 116:1881–1893

274. Munhoz AM, Ishida LH, Sturtz GP et al (2004) Importance of lateral row perforator vessels in deep inferior epigastric perforator flap harvesting. Plast Reconstr Surg 113:517–524

275. Murakami R, Fujii T, Itoh T et al (1996) Versatility of the thin groin flap. Microsurgery 17:41–47

276. Murphy JB (1897) Resection of arteries and veins injured in continuity-end-to-end suture: experimental and clinical research. Med Rec 51:73

277. Myong CP (1986) An anatomic study of the radial collateral branch of deep brachial artery. PhD dissertation, University of Seoul

278. Nakajima H, Fujino T, Adachi S (1986) A new concept of vascular supply to the skin and classification of skin flaps according to their vascularization. Ann Plast Surg 16:1–19

279. Nassif TM, Mayer B, Bijos PB (1988) [The parascapular cutaneous latissimus dorsi osteomyocutaneous double flap. Free monobloc transfer in facial reconstruction]. Chirurg 59:793–796

280. Nassif TM, Vidal L, Bovet JL et al (1982) The parascapular flap: a new cutaneous microsurgical free flap. Plast Reconstr Surg 69:591–600

281. Neligan PC, Blondeel PN, Morris SF et al (2005) Perforator flaps: overview, classification and nomenclature. In Blondeel PN, Hallock GG, Morris SF et al (eds) Perforator Flaps: Anatomy, Technique and Clinical Applications. Quality Medical Publishing, Inc, St. Louis, pp 37–52

282. Nincovic M (2005) Superficial inferior epigastric artery perforator. In Blondeel PN, Hallock GG, Morris SF et al (eds) Perforator Flaps: Anatomy, Technique and Clinical Applications. Quality Medical Publishing, Inc., St. Louis, pp 405–420

283. Niranjan NS, Watson DP (1990) Reconstruction of the cheek using a "suspended" radial forearm free flap. Br J Plast Surg 43:365–366

284. Nojima K, Brown SA, Acikel C et al (2005) Defining vascular supply and territory of thinned perforator flaps: part I. Anterolateral thigh perforator flap. Plast Reconstr Surg 116:182–193

285. Nylen CD (1924) An oto-microscope. Acta Otolaryngol 5:414

286. O'Brien B, Morrison WA (1987) Reconstructive microsurgery. Churchhill, Livingston

287. Olivari N (1976) The latissimus flap. Br J Plast Surg 29:126–128

288. Orticochea M (1972) A new method of total reconstruction of the penis. Br J Plast Surg 25:347–366

289. Ostrup LT, Fredrickson JM (1974) Distant transfer of a free, living bone graft by microvascular anastomoses. An experimental study. Plast Reconstr Surg 54:274–285

290. Parrett BM, Caterson SA, Tobias AM et al (2008) DIEP flaps in women with abdominal scars: are complication rates affected? Plast Reconstr Surg 121:1527–1531

291. Patel SA, Keller A (2008) A theoretical model describing arterial flow in the DIEP flap related to number and size of perforator vessels. J Plast Reconstr Aesthet Surg 61:1316–1320; discussion 1320

292. Pennington DG, Pelly AD (1980) The rectus abdominis myocutaneous free flap. Br J Plast Surg 33:277–282

293. Pennington DG, Nettle WJ, Lam P (1993) Microvascular augmentation of the blood supply of the contralateral side of the free transverse rectus abdominis musculocutaneous flap. Ann Plast Surg 31:123–126; discussion 126–127

294. Pistner H, Reuther J, Bill J (1990) [The scapula region as a potential donor area for microsurgical transplants]. Fortschr Kiefer Gesichtschir 35:87–90

295. Porter CJ, Mellow CG (2001) Anatomically aberrant forearm arteries: an absent radial artery with co-dominant median and ulnar arteries. Br J Plast Surg 54:727–728

296. Posch NA, Mureau MA, Flood SJ et al (2005) The combined free partial vastus lateralis with anterolateral thigh perforator flap reconstruction of extensive composite defects. Br J Plast Surg 58:1095–1103

297. Pribaz JJ, Orgill DP, Epstein MD et al (1995) Anterolateral thigh free flap. Ann Plast Surg 34:585–592

298. Quain R (1844) Anatomy of the arteries of the human body. Taylor and Walton, London

299. Quillen CG (1979) Latissimus dorsi myocutaneous flaps in head and neck reconstruction. Plast Reconstr Surg 63:664–670

300. Quillen CG, Shearin JC Jr, Georgiade NG (1978) Use of the latissimus dorsi myocutaneous island flap for reconstruction in the head and neck area: case report. Plast Reconstr Surg 62:113–117

301. Rajacic N, Gang RK, Krishnan J et al (2002) Thin anterolateral thigh free flap. Ann Plast Surg 48:252–257

302. Ramasastry SS, Tucker JB, Swartz WM et al (1984) The internal oblique muscle flap: an anatomic and clinical study. Plast Reconstr Surg 73:721–733

303. Rand RP, Cramer MM, Strandness DE Jr (1994) Color-flow duplex scanning in the preoperative assessment of TRAM flap perforators: a report of 32 consecutive patients. Plast Reconstr Surg 93:453–459

304. Reinert S (2000) The free revascularized lateral upper arm flap in maxillofacial reconstruction following ablative tumour surgery. J Craniomaxillofac Surg 28:69–73

305. Reuther J (1992) Surgical therapy of oral carcinomas. J Craniomaxillofac Surg 20:24

306. Ribuffo D, Cigna E, Gargano F et al (2005) The innervated anterolateral thigh flap: anatomical study and clinical implications. Plast Reconstr Surg 115:464–470

307. Riediger D (1983) Mikrochirurgische Weichgewebstransplantate in die Gesichtsregion. Hanser, Munich

308. Riediger D (1988) Restoration of masticatory function by microsurgically revascularized iliac crest bone grafts using enosseous implants. Plast Reconstr Surg 81:861–877

309. Riediger D, Schmelzle R (1986) [Modified use of the myocutaneous latissimus dorsi flap for repairing defects in the oral and maxillofacial region]. Dtsch Z Mund Kiefer Gesichtschir 10:364–374

310. Riediger D, Ehrenfeld M (1990) Mikrochirurgischer Weichgewebstransfer in die Mund-Kiefer-Gesichtsregion. In Schuchardt K (ed) Fortschritte in der Kiefer- und Gesichtschirurgie. Thieme, Stuttgart

311. Rivet D, Buffet M, Martin D et al (1987) The lateral arm flap: an anatomic study. J Reconstr Microsurg 3:121–132

312. Robson MC, Zachary LS, Schmidt DR et al (1989) Reconstruction of large cranial defects in the presence of heavy radiation damage and infection utilizing tissue transferred by microvascular anastomoses. Plast Reconstr Surg 83:438–442

313. Rojviroj S, Mahaisavariya B, Sirichativapee W et al (1989) Vastus lateralis myocutaneous flap: the treatment for trochanteric pressure sores in paraplegic patient. J Med Assoc Thai 72:629–632

314. Romanes GJ (1981) Cunningham's textbook of anatomy, 12th edn. Oxford University Press, Oxford

315. Ross GL, Dunn R, Kirkpatrick J et al (2003) To thin or not to thin: the use of the anterolateral thigh flap in the reconstruction of intraoral defects. Br J Plast Surg 56:409–413

316. Rowsell AR, Godfrey AM, Richards MA (1986) The thinned latissimus dorsi free flap: a case report. Br J Plast Surg 39:210–212

317. Rowsell AR, Davies DM, Eisenberg N et al (1984) The anatomy of the subscapular-thoracodorsal arterial system: study of 100 cadaver dissections. Br J Plast Surg 37:574–576

318. Rowsell AR, Eisenberg N, Davies DM et al (1986) The anatomy of the thoracodorsal artery within the latissimus dorsi muscle. Br J Plast Surg 39:206–209

319. Rozen WM, Tran TM, Ashton MW et al (2008) Refining the course of the thoracolumbar nerves: a new understanding of the innervation of the anterior abdominal wall. Clin Anat 21:325–333

320. Rozen WM, Ribuffo D, Atzeni M et al (2009) Current state of the art in perforator flap imaging with computed tomographic angiography. Surg Radiol Anat 31:631–639

321. Russell RC, Pribaz J, Zook EG et al (1986) Functional evaluation of latissimus dorsi donor site. Plast Reconstr Surg 78:336–344

322. Sadove RC, Merrell JC (1987) The split rectus abdominis free muscle transfer. Ann Plast Surg 18:179–181

323. Sadove RC, Luce EA, McGrath PC (1991) Reconstruction of the lower lip and chin with the composite radial forearm-palmaris longus free flap. Plast Reconstr Surg 88:209–214

324. Sadove RC, Sengezer M, McRoberts JW et al (1993) One-stage total penile reconstruction with a free sensate osteocutaneous fibula flap. Plast Reconstr Surg 92:1314–1323; discussion 1324–1325

325. Safak T, Akyurek M (2000) Free transfer of the radial forearm flap with preservation of the radial artery. Ann Plast Surg 45:97–99

326. Saijo M (1978) The vascular territories of the dorsal trunk: a reappraisal for potential flap donor sites. Br J Plast Surg 31:200–204

327. Saint-Cyr M, Schaverien MV, Rohrich RJ (2009) Perforator flaps: history, controversies, physiology, anatomy, and use in reconstruction. Plast Reconstr Surg 123:132e–145e

328. Salibian AH, Tesoro VR, Wood DL (1983) Staged transfer of a free microvascular latissimus dorsi myocutaneous flap using saphenous vein grafts. Plast Reconstr Surg 71:543–547

329. Sanders R, Mayou BJ (1979) A new vascularized bone graft transferred by microvascular anastomosis as a free flap. Br J Surg 66:787–788

330. Santanelli F, Paolini G, Renzi L (2008) Preliminary experience in breast reconstruction with the free vertical deep inferior epigastric perforator flap. Scand J Plast Reconstr Surg Hand Surg 42:23–27

331. Sasaki K, Nozaki M, Aiba H et al (2000) A rare variant of the radial artery: clinical considerations in raising a radial forearm flap. Br J Plast Surg 53:445–447

332. Satoh K, Yoshikawa A, Hayashi M (1988) Reverse-flow anterior tibial flap type III. Br J Plast Surg 41:624–627

333. Satoh K, Ohkubo F, Tojima Y (1991) A variation of the vascular pedicle of the latissimus dorsi muscle. Plast Reconstr Surg 88:1081–1084

334. Satoh K, Le Danvic M, Matsui A et al (1988) [Peroneal flaps with or without vascularized fibular bone graft in reconstructions of the lower limb]. Ann Chir Plast Esthet 33:119–126

335. Schaverien M, Saint-Cyr M, Arbique G et al (2008) Arterial and venous anatomies of the deep inferior epigastric perforator and superficial inferior epigastric artery flaps. Plast Reconstr Surg 121:1909–1919

336. Schaverien M, Saint-Cyr M, Arbique G et al (2008) Three- and four-dimensional computed tomographic angiography and venography of the anterolateral thigh perforator flap. Plast Reconstr Surg 121:1685–1696

337. Schaverien MV, Perks AG, McCulley SJ (2007) Comparison of outcomes and donor-site morbidity in unilateral free TRAM versus DIEP flap breast reconstruction. J Plast Reconstr Aesthet Surg 60:1219–1224

338. Scheker LR, Kleinert HE, Hanel DP (1987) Lateral arm composite tissue transfer to ipsilateral hand defects. J Hand Surg Am 12:665–672

339. Schlenz I, Korak KJ, Kunstfeld R et al (2001) The dermis-prelaminated scapula flap for reconstructions of the hard palate and the alveolar ridge: a clinical and histologic evaluation. Plast Reconstr Surg 108:1519–1524; discussion 1525–1526

340. Schmelzle R (1986) [Vascular pedicled iliac crest transplant and its use in the jaw]. Handchir Mikrochir Plast Chir 18:376–378

341. Schoeller T, Wechselberger G, Roger J et al (2007) Management of infraumbilical vertical scars in DIEP-flaps by crossover anastomosis. J Plast Reconstr Aesthet Surg 60:524–528

342. Schoofs M, Millot F, Patenotre P et al (1988) [The peroneal flap: its value in distal covering of the lower limbs]. Ann Chir Plast Esthet 33:273–276

343. Schusterman MA, Reece GP, Miller MJ et al (1992) The osteocutaneous free fibula flap: is the skin paddle reliable? Plast Reconstr Surg 90:787–793; discussion 794–798

344. Schustermann MA, Acland RD, Banis JC et al (1983) The lateral arm flap: an experimental and clinical study. In Williams HC (ed) Transactions of the VIII International Congress of Plastic Surgery, Montreal

345. Seidenberg B, Rosenak SS, Hurwitt ES et al (1959) Immediate reconstruction of the cervical esophagus by a revascularized isolated jejunal segment. Ann Surg 149:162–171

231

346. Seitz A, Papp S, Papp C et al (1999) The anatomy of the angular branch of the thoracodorsal artery. Cells Tissues Organs 164:227–236

347. Sekido M, Yamamoto Y, Makino S (2006) Maxillary reconstruction using a free deep inferior epigastric perforator (DIEP) flap combined with vascularised costal cartilages. J Plast Reconstr Aesthet Surg 59:1350–1354

348. Sekiguchi J, Kobayashi S, Ohmori K (1993) Use of the osteocutaneous free scapular flap on the lower extremities. Plast Reconstr Surg 91:103–112

349. Serra JM, Paloma V, Mesa F et al (1991) The vascularized fibula graft in mandibular reconstruction. J Oral Maxillofac Surg 49:244–250

350. Shaw WW, Hidalgo DA (1987) Microsurgery in trauma. Futura Publishing, Mount Kisco, New York

351. Shenaq SM (1987) Pretransfer expansion of a sensate lateral arm free flap. Ann Plast Surg 19:558–562

352. Shesol BF, Clarke JS (1980) Intrathoracic application of the latissimus dorsi musculocutaneous flap. Plast Reconstr Surg 66:842–845

353. Shestak KC, Schusterman MA, Jones NF et al (1988) Immediate microvascular reconstruction of combined palatal and midfacial defects using soft tissue only. Microsurgery 9:128–131

354. Shieh SJ, Chiu HY, Yu JC et al (2000) Free anterolateral thigh flap for reconstruction of head and neck defects following cancer ablation. Plast Reconstr Surg 105:2349–2357; discussion 2358–2360

355. Shindo M, Fong BP, Funk GF et al (2000) The fibula osteocutaneous flap in head and neck reconstruction: a critical evaluation of donor site morbidity. Arch Otolaryngol Head Neck Surg 126:1467–1472

356. Silverberg B, Banis JC Jr, Acland RD (1985) Mandibular reconstruction with microvascular bone transfer. Series of 10 patients. Am J Surg 150:440–446

357. Silverton JS, Nahai F, Jurkiewicz MJ (1978) The latissimus dorsi myocutaneous flap to replace a defect on the upper arm. Br J Plast Surg 31:29–31

358. Small JO, Millar R (1985) The radial artery forearm flap: an anomaly of the radial artery. Br J Plast Surg 38:501–503

359. Song R, Song Y, Yu Y (1982) The upper arm free flap. Clin Plast Surg 9:27–35

360. Song R, Gao Y, Song Y et al (1982) The forearm flap. Clin Plast Surg 9:21–26

361. Song YG, Chen GZ, Song YL (1984) The free thigh flap: a new free flap concept based on the septocutaneous artery. Br J Plast Surg 37:149–159

362. Soutar DS, Tanner NS (1984) The radial forearm flap in the management of soft tissue injuries of the hand. Br J Plast Surg 37:18–26

363. Soutar DS, Widdowson WP (1986) Immediate reconstruction of the mandible using a vascularized segment of radius. Head Neck Surg 8:232–246

364. Soutar DS, McGregor IA (1986) The radial forearm flap in intraoral reconstruction: the experience of 60 consecutive cases. Plast Reconstr Surg 78:1–8

365. Soutar DS, Scheker LR, Tanner NS et al (1983) The radial forearm flap: a versatile method for intra-oral reconstruction. Br J Plast Surg 36:1–8

366. Spateholz W (1893) Die Verheilung der Blutgefäße in der Haut. Arch Anat Physiol 1:1

367. Stock W, Stock M (1983) Der osteokutane Unterarmlappen. Handchir 15:49

368. Stranc MF, Globerman DY (1989) Accidental reinnervation as a complication of latissimus dorsi free flap to the face and scalp. Br J Plast Surg 42:341–343

369. Strauch B, Yu G (1993) Atlas of microvascular surgery. Thieme, New York

370. Swanson E, Boyd JB, Manktelow RT (1990) The radial forearm flap: reconstructive applications and donor-site defects in 35 consecutive patients. Plast Reconstr Surg 85:258–266

371. Swartz WM, Ramasastry SS, McGill JR et al (1987) Distally based vastus lateralis muscle flap for coverage of wounds about the knee. Plast Reconstr Surg 80:255–265

372. Swartz WM, Banis JC, Newton ED et al (1986) The osteocutaneous scapular flap for mandibular and maxillary reconstruction. Plast Reconstr Surg 77:530–545

373. Takada K, Sugata T, Yoshiga K et al (1987) Total upper lip reconstruction using a free radial forearm flap incorporating the brachioradialis muscle: report of a case. J Oral Maxillofac Surg 45:959–962

374. Tan O (2009) Versatility of the vertical designed deep inferior epigastric perforator flap. Microsurgery 29:282–286

375. Tang M, Mao Y, Almutairi K et al (2009) Three-dimensional analysis of perforators of the posterior leg. Plast Reconstr Surg 123:1729–1738

376. Tansatit T, Wanidchaphloi S, Sanguansit P (2008) The anatomy of the lateral circumflex femoral artery in anterolateral thigh flap. J Med Assoc Thai 91:1404–1409

377. Tansini I (1896) Nuovo processo per l' amputazione della mammaella per cancere. Riforma Med 12:3

378. Taylor GI (1982) Reconstruction of the mandible with free composite iliac bone grafts. Ann Plast Surg 9:361–376

379. Taylor GI (1983) The current status of free vascularized bone grafts. Clin Plast Surg 10:185–209

380. Taylor GI (2003) The angiosomes of the body and their supply to perforator flaps. Clin Plast Surg 30:331–342

381. Taylor GI, Daniel RK (1975) The anatomy of several free flap donor sites. Plast Reconstr Surg 56:243–253

382. Taylor GI, Miller GD, Ham FJ (1975) The free vascularized bone graft. A clinical extension of microvascular techniques. Plast Reconstr Surg 55:533–544

383. Taylor GI, Townsend P, Corlett R (1979) Superiority of the deep circumflex iliac vessels as the supply for free groin flaps. Plast Reconstr Surg 64:595–604

384. Taylor GI, Corlett RJ, Boyd JB (1984) The versatile deep inferior epigastric (inferior rectus abdominis) flap. Br J Plast Surg 37:330–350

385. Taylor GI, Caddy CM, Watterson PA et al (1990) The venous territories (venosomes) of the human body: experimental study and clinical implications. Plast Reconstr Surg 86:185–213

386. Teot L, Bosse JP, Moufarrage R et al (1981) The scapular crest pedicled bone graft. Int J Microsurg 3:257

387. Thoma A, Archibald S, Jackson S et al (1994) Surgical patterns of venous drainage of the free forearm flap in head and neck reconstruction. Plast Reconstr Surg 93:54–59

388. Timmons MJ (1984) William Harvey revisited: reverse flow through the valves of forearm veins. Lancet 2:394–395

389. Timmons MJ, Missotten FE, Poole MD et al (1986) Complications of radial forearm flap donor sites. Br J Plast Surg 39:176–178

390. Tobin GR, Schusterman M, Peterson GH et al (1981) The intramuscular neurovascular anatomy of the latissimus dorsi muscle: the basis for splitting the flap. Plast Reconstr Surg 67:637–641

391. Tolhurst DE, Haeseker B (1982) Fasciocutaneous flaps in the axillary region. Br J Plast Surg 35:430–435

392. Tran NV, Buchel EW, Convery PA (2007) Microvascular complications of DIEP flaps. Plast Reconstr Surg 119:1397–405; discussion 1406–408

393. Tsai FC, Yang JY, Chuang SS et al (2002) Combined method of free lateral leg perforator flap with cervicoplasty for reconstruction of anterior cervical scar contractures: a new flap. J Reconstr Microsurg 18:185–190

394. Tsai FC, Yang JY, Mardini S et al (2004) Free split-cutaneous perforator flaps procured using a three-dimensional harvest technique for the reconstruction of post-burn contracture defects. Plast Reconstr Surg 113:185–193; discussion 194–195

395. Tsukino A, Kurachi K, Inamiya T et al (2004) Preoperative color Doppler assessment in planning of anterolateral thigh flaps. Plast Reconstr Surg 113:241–246

396. Upton J, Albin RE, Mulliken JB et al (1992) The use of scapular and parascapular flaps for cheek reconstruction. Plast Reconstr Surg 90:959–971

397. Urbaniak JR, Koman LA, Goldner RD et al (1982) The vascularized cutaneous scapular flap. Plast Reconstr Surg 69:772–778

398. Urken ML (1992) Discussion. The osteocutaneous free fibula flap: is the skin paddle reliable? Plast Reconstr Surg 90:787

399. Urken ML, Cheney ML, Sullivan MJ et al (1990) Atlas of regional and free flaps for head and neck reconstruction. Raven Press, New York

400. Urken ML, Weinberg H, Vickery C et al (1990) The neurofasciocutaneous radial forearm flap in head and neck reconstruction: a preliminary report. Laryngoscope 100:161–173

401. Urken ML, Vickery C, Weinberg H et al (1989) The internal oblique-iliac crest osseomyocutaneous microvascular free flap in head and neck reconstruction. J Reconstr Microsurg 5:203–214; discussion 215–216

402. Urken ML, Turk JB, Weinberg H et al (1991) The rectus abdominis free flap in head and neck reconstruction. Arch Otolaryngol Head Neck Surg 117:1031

403. Urken ML, Vickery C, Weinberg H et al (1989) The internal oblique-iliac crest osseomyocutaneous free flap in oromandibular reconstruction. Report of 20 cases. Arch Otolaryngol Head Neck Surg 115:339–349

404. Urken ML, Catalano PJ, Sen C et al (1993) Free tissue transfer for skull base reconstruction analysis of complications and a classification scheme for defining skull base defects. Arch Otolaryngol Head Neck Surg 119:1318–1325

405. Urken ML, Weinberg H, Buchbinder D et al (1994) Microvascular free flaps in head and neck reconstruction. Report of 200 cases and review of complications. Arch Otolaryngol Head Neck Surg 120:633–640

406. van Twisk R, Pavlov PW, Sonneveld J (1988) Reconstruction of bone and soft tissue defects with free fibula transfer. Ann Plast Surg 21:555–558

407. Vandevoort M, Vranckx JJ, Fabre G (2002) Perforator topography of the deep inferior epigastric perforator flap in 100 cases of breast reconstruction. Plast Reconstr Surg 109:1912–1918

408. Verpaele AM, Blondeel PN, Van Landuyt K et al (1999) The superior gluteal artery perforator flap: an additional tool in the treatment of sacral pressure sores. Br J Plast Surg 52:385–391

409. Villaret DB, Futran NA (2003) The indications and outcomes in the use of osteocutaneous radial forearm free flap. Head Neck 25:475–481

410. von Lanz T, Wachsmuth W (1972) Teil 4: Bein und Statik, 2nd edn. Springer-Verlag, Berlin Heidelberg New York

411. Vyas RM, Dickinson BP, Fastekjian JH et al (2008) Risk factors for abdominal donor-site morbidity in free flap breast reconstruction. Plast Reconstr Surg 121:1519–1526

412. Waterhouse N, Healy C (1990) The versatility of the lateral arm flap. Br J Plast Surg 43:398–402

413. Watson JS, Craig RD, Orton CI (1979) The free latissimus dorsi myocutaneous flap. Plast Reconstr Surg 64:299–305

414. Weber RA, Pederson WC (1995) Skin paddle salvage in the fibula osteocutaneous free flap with secondary skin paddle vascular anastomosis. J Reconstr Microsurg 11:239–241; discussion 242–244

415. Wee JT (1986) Reconstruction of the lower leg and foot with the reverse-pedicled anterior tibial flap: preliminary report of a new fasciocutaneous flap. Br J Plast Surg 39:327–337

416. Wei FC, Chen HC, Chuang CC et al (1986) Fibular osteoseptocutaneous flap: anatomic study and clinical application. Plast Reconstr Surg 78:191–200

417. Wei FC, Jain V, Suominen S et al (2001) Confusion among perforator flaps: what is a true perforator flap? Plast Reconstr Surg 107:874–876

418. Wei FC, Seah CS, Tsai YC et al (1994) Fibula osteoseptocutaneous flap for reconstruction of composite mandibular defects. Plast Reconstr Surg 93:294–304; discussion 305–306

419. Wei FC, Jain V, Celik N et al (2002) Have we found an ideal soft-tissue flap? An experience with 672 anterolateral thigh flaps. Plast Reconstr Surg 109:2219–2226; discussion 2227–2230

420. Williams LP, Warwick R (1980) Grey's Anatomy, 36th edn. Churchill Livingston, Edinburgh

421. Wolff KD (1993) The supramalleolar flap based on septocutaneous perforators from the peroneal vessels for intraoral soft tissue replacement. Br J Plast Surg 46:151–155

422. Wolff KD (1998) Indications for the vastus lateralis flap in oral and maxillofacial surgery. Br J Oral Maxillofac Surg 36:358–364

423. Wolff KD, Metelmann HR (1992) Applications of the lateral vastus muscle flap. Int J Oral Maxillofac Surg 21:215–218

424. Wolff KD, Grundmann A (1992) The free vastus lateralis flap: an anatomic study with case reports. Plast Reconstr Surg 89:469–475; discussion 476–477

425. Wolff KD, Stellmach R (1995) The osteoseptocutaneous or purely septocutaneous peroneal flap with a supramalleolar skin paddle. Int J Oral Maxillofac Surg 24:38–43

426. Wolff KD, Howaldt HP (1995) Three years of experience with the free vastus lateralis flap: an analysis of 30 consecutive reconstructions in maxillofacial surgery. Ann Plast Surg 34:35–42

427. Wolff KD, Dienemann D, Hoffmeister B (1995) Intraoral defect coverage with muscle flaps. J Oral Maxillofac Surg 53:680–685; discussion 686

428. Wolff KD, Ervens J, Hoffmeister B (1996) Improvement of the radial forearm donor site by prefabrication of fascial-split-thickness skin grafts. Plast Reconstr Surg 98:358–362

429. Wolff KD, Plath T, Hoffmeister B (2000) Primary thinning of the myocutaneous vastus lateralis flap. Int J Oral Maxillofac Surg 29:272–276

430. Wolff KD, Hölzle F, Nolte D (2004) Perforator flaps from the lateral lower leg for intraoral reconstruction. Plast Reconstr Surg 113:107–113

431. Wolff KD, Ervens J, Herzog K et al (1996) Experience with the osteocutaneous fibula flap: an analysis of 24 consecutive reconstructions of composite mandibular defects. J Craniomaxillofac Surg 24:330–338

432. Wolff KD, Plath T, Frege J et al (2000) [Primary thinning and de-epithelialization of microsurgical transplants from the lateral thigh]. Mund Kiefer Gesichtschir 4:88–94

433. Wolff KD, Kesting M, Löffelbein D et al (2007) Perforator-based anterolateral thigh adipofascial or dermal fat flaps for facial contour augmentation. J Reconstr Microsurg 23:497–503

434. Wolff KD, Kesting M, Thurmuller P et al (2006) The early use of a perforator flap of the lateral lower limb in maxillofacial reconstructive surgery. Int J Oral Maxillofac Surg 35:602–607

435. Wong CH, Tan BK, Wei FC et al (2007) Use of the soleus musculocutaneous perforator for skin paddle salvage of the fibula osteoseptocutaneous flap: anatomical study and clinical confirmation. Plast Reconstr Surg 120:1576–1584

436. Wong CH, Wei FC, Fu B et al (2009) Alternative vascular pedicle of the anterolateral thigh flap: the oblique branch of the lateral circumflex femoral artery. Plast Reconstr Surg 123:571–577

437. Wu LC, Bajaj A, Chang DW et al (2008) Comparison of donor-site morbidity of SIEA, DIEP, and muscle-sparing TRAM flaps for breast reconstruction. Plast Reconstr Surg 122:702–709

438. Yamada A, Harii K, Ueda K et al (1992) Free rectus abdominis muscle reconstruction of the anterior skull base. Br J Plast Surg 45:302–306

439. Yamada A, Harii K, Itoh Y et al (1993) Reconstruction of the cervical trachea with a free forearm flap. Br J Plast Surg 46:32–35

440. Yang G, Chen B, Gao Y et al (1981) Forearm free skin transplantation. Nat Med J China 61:139

441. Yang JY, Tsai FC, Chana JS et al (2002) Use of free thin anterolateral thigh flaps combined with cervicoplasty for reconstruction of postburn anterior cervical contractures. Plast Reconstr Surg 110:39–46

442. Yang WG, Chiang YC, Wei FC et al (2006) Thin anterolateral thigh perforator flap using a modified perforator microdissection technique and its clinical application for foot resurfacing. Plast Reconstr Surg 117:1004–1008

443. Yano T, Sakuraba M, Asano T et al (2009) Head and neck reconstruction with the deep inferior epigastric perforator flap: a report of two cases. Microsurgery 29:287–292

235

444. Yokoo S, Komori T, Furudoi S et al (2001) Rare variant of the intrasoleus musculo-cutaneous perforator: clinical considerations in raising a free peroneal osteocutaneous flap. J Reconstr Microsurg 17:225–228

445. Yoshimura M, Shimada T, Hosokawa M (1990) The vasculature of the peroneal tissue transfer. Plast Reconstr Surg 85:917–921

446. Yoshimura M, Imura S, Shimamura K et al (1984) Peroneal flap for reconstruction in the extremity: preliminary report. Plast Reconstr Surg 74:402–409

447. Yoshimura M, Shimada T, Matsuda M et al (1989) Double peroneal free flap for multiple skin defects of the hand. Br J Plast Surg 42:715–718

448. Yu P, Youssef A (2006) Efficacy of the handheld Doppler in preoperative identification of the cutaneous perforators in the anterolateral thigh flap. Plast Reconstr Surg 118:928–933; discussion 934–935

449. Zhang SC (1983) [Clinical application of medial skin flap of leg – analysis of 9 cases]. Zhonghua Wai Ke Za Zhi 21:743–45

450. Zhou G, Qiao Q, Chen GY et al (1991) Clinical experience and surgical anatomy of 32 free anterolateral thigh flap transplantations. Br J Plast Surg 44:91–96

451. Zhou Y, Chen L, Hu S et al (2002) Brachial plexus injury after transfer of free latissimus dorsi musculocutaneous flap. Chin J Traumatol 5:254–256

Subject Index

239